Y0-ABS-763

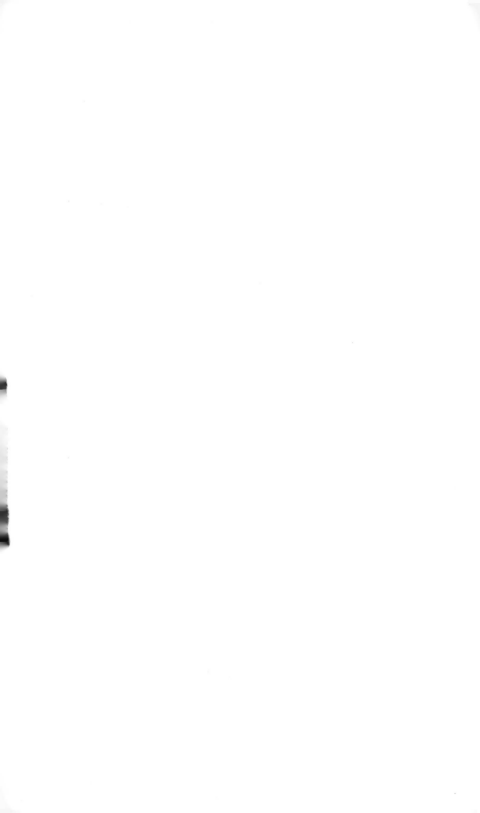

Clinical Practice
In
Community
Mental Health
Centers

H. G. WHITTINGTON, M.D.

Clinical Practice
In
Community
Mental Health
Centers

INTERNATIONAL UNIVERSITIES
PRESS, INC.   New York

Library of Congress Catalog Card Number: 77–18441
ISBN: 0–8236–0955–3

Manufactured in the United States of America

Contents

CHAPTER I

The Comprehensive Community Mental Health Center

THE COMMUNITY mental health center is an innovative service delivery system, made necessary by the development in the United States of multiple service systems which proved inefficient, segregated, uncomprehensive, and exclusivistic. The mental health center is an attempt, then, to reconcile and reunite disparate approaches in the applied behavioral sciences.

The mental health center stands in relation to preexisting service delivery systems as a supermarket does to the corner grocery, the department store to the specialty shop. It opens new opportunities for patients and staff alike and places new responsibilities upon the staff. No longer must the individual clinician know only his product or service; he must also be aware of the full range of offerings available within the comprehensive community mental health center, indeed within the total community, and must serve not only as treator but also as broker, helping obtain needed services for the patient.

President Kennedy's message to Congress (1963), and subsequent legislation and regulations which launched the National Community Mental Health Centers program, clearly contemplated primarily a mental *illness* center. Congress was told that patients could be treated in their home communities, that the population of state hospitals could be reduced 50 per cent in 10 years, that treatment could be financed largely through third-party payment systems, and that psychiatry could be returned to the mainstream of American medicine. Our word magic—in calling such enterprises mental *health* centers—has resulted in confusion among the applied behavioral science professions and a lack of consensus about the legitimate domain of the center. This semantic inexactness, however, has not confused our constituency at all: The ill, distressed, unhappy, and pained flock to community mental health centers expecting mental illness services in the form of diagnosis, treatment, and relief of symptoms.

This book is designed as a primer of clinical practice in such comprehensive community mental health centers. It considers the work of the community mental health center, its new opportunities and unique requirements, and explores the application of standard psychiatric practice in this new context.

Certain basic principles underlie the clinical program of the comprehensive community mental health center. These concepts are expressed in the regulations governing the administration of construction and staffing funds by the National Institute of Mental Health. These ideas strongly influence clinical practice and require preliminary discussion:

1. Each center serves a circumscribed population

group, defined as individuals living in a contiguous area in which the center is located. The National Institute of Mental Health regulations have arbitrarily defined the minimum size of the population to be served as 75,000, the maximum size as 200,000. The intent of this regulation, reflecting as it does service patterns in England, Russia, and other advanced nations, is to insure accountability within the public sector, in order to advance the other aims of the comprehensive community mental health center elaborated below. The premise is that all citizens living within the catchment area of the center will have unrestricted access to all of the services of the center, and that this will serve to avoid "shopping trips" by patients to find adequate care. The catchment area concept does not imply that an individual living within a particular center's catchment area will be forced to use that center, nor in any way is the concept to vitiate choice of treator by the patient or prospective patient. Rather, it is an administrative arrangement designed to insure accountability on the part of the community mental health center.

2. Comprehensiveness of service receives great emphasis in community mental health center planning. Fragmentation of services in this country has created great difficulty for patients. Particular clinical facilities have provided only a few specific treatment services, requiring the patient to go through a laborious process to find the appropriate facility affording the needed service. Agencies providing only a few services are also not well suited to meet the needs of the chronically and seriously ill, whose ser-

vice requirements characteristically shift during their longitudinal treatment careers.

The National Institute of Mental Health has defined by regulation five essential elements of service necessary to insure comprehensiveness: (a) Outpatient services, (b) 24-hour hospitalization services, (c) Partial hospitalization services, (d) Emergency psychiatric services, and (e) Consultation and education services. In addition, NIMH defines other desirable elements of service that should be available if the ideal of true comprehensiveness is to be achieved: (a) Training and education, (b) Research, (c) Rehabilitation, (d) Precare and aftercare, and (e) Special diagnostic and other services.

3. Continuity of care has been sadly lacking on the American psychiatric scene. Discontinuity has been evident as patients move from one system to another—such as from the private practice system to the state hospital system, from the community psychiatric clinic to the state hospital, and so forth. Discontinuity has also been rampant in most public psychiatric facilities: The patient characteristically had multiple primary clinicians as he moved through the treatment program. It is the intent of the comprehensive community mental health center to minimize discontinuities in treatment, both in administrative auspices and in terms of the primary clinician involved. This places additional demands upon the clinician in the comprehensive center, both technically and psychologically: No longer can he play the game of "passing the buck," moving the patient on to some unsuspecting colleague or some quite separate clinical element. He is expected,

wherever humanely feasible, to maintain primary responsibility as his patient moves through a treatment career. This concept of continuity also casts the psychiatric team in an entirely new light, since in the past the traditional psychiatric team has often served to covertly fragment responsibility for care.

4. Availability of service is an extremely important consideration in designing a community mental health center program. There are a number of dimensions of availability:

a. Geographic availability implies that services should be decentralized within the neighborhood, readily available on foot and by public transportation. Where necessary, service should be deployed to the patient's home.

b. Temporal availability means the patient should be seen promptly upon application for service, not delayed or placed on a waiting list. Service should be available at times when it is feasible for the patient to abandon other role commitments in order to visit the facility.

c. Financial availability implies a flexible fee-setting policy which allows indigent or low income patients to receive service below cost or without charge. There is no convincing evidence that free service is less effectively utilized than expensive care.

d. Social availability necessitates an extensive community education program to change attitudes within the community about mental illness and the seeking of psychiatric help. Without such efforts, stigmatization arising from psychiatric treatment results in unnecessary and damaging delays in seeking clinical assistance, since the prospective patient fears rejection by his family and community.

The National Mental Health Plan calls for the establishment of 2,000 comprehensive community mental health centers in the United States by approximately 1980, each of which will conform to the pattern described above. It is clear that this numerical goal will not be reached or even approximated. It is hoped that in addition to care that is readily available, comprehensive and continuous, deployed in a defined geographic area and directed towards a specific population, many of these centers will also be characterized by high quality clinical service. Our preoccupation with organizational and administrative details has temporarily turned our professional attention away from issues of quality. The author hopes this book will focus attention on maintenance of high standards of clinical care as a major responsibility of the mental health professions in this new endeavor.

In deciding how to achieve quality in the clinical program, a *systems* stance must also be maintained if we are to make rational decisions about how best to deploy our professional resources and are to decide as individual professionals how most usefully to deploy our talents and energy. By adopting this focus, the community psychiatrist perhaps departs most radically from the traditional clinical practitioner whose attention is almost exclusively upon the individual patient. In designing and implementing a community mental health program, the community psychiatrist must also be concerned with other issues.

An initial consideration is how to evaluate the

effectiveness of a community mental health program. Effectiveness may be viewed as a function of utilization, patient characteristics, and the services offered. To discuss each in turn:

1. *Utilization.* If the community mental health practitioner is to be concerned about the impact of his program upon the psychiatric morbidity of a population-at-risk, he must study his center's utilization rate. To the extent that we believe our change technology is useful and successful in reducing morbidity in the psychiatrically ill individuals who receive treatment, we must attempt to attain a high utilization rate. A low utilization rate with prolonged treatment careers might produce excellent results in terms of the before treatment/after treatment differences in patients receiving the service. A clinical program that offered service to four times as many patients, however, while having a less marked before treatment/after treatment difference in individual patients, might be a much more effective clinical service from the standpoint of the community.

There are obviously clear limits in pressing the maximum utilization model to its logical extreme. Any center has fixed resources, which are never fully adequate to meet the demand for service from the community. It is characteristic of our society that demand increases more rapidly than resources to meet that demand, no matter what the product or service. The community mental health practitioner, then, will usually be in the position of artificially limiting the utilization of his service to some extent, so that his personnel and clinical capabilities are not impossibly overtaxed. Usually, when he must answer the question, "Shall I treat this case for one year, with a questionable outcome; or shall I treat these four other cases for three months each, with a moderately successful outcome?", he will elect to treat four cases briefly rather than one case over a prolonged period of time. These are the hard decisions that must be made by a professional mental health worker faced with the mass casualty situation that characterizes psychiatric morbidity in the United States today. It is not a pleasant task; it is a task with major ethical dilemmas and a responsibility that must be shouldered by the practitioner, rather than leaving it to chance. Giving optimum service to the people who come first to the center while leaving the unlucky latecomers to languish on the waiting list and to get little or no service is reprehensible to the author, persisting only because it is a "cop out" which allows the practitioner to avoid making the hard decisions of responsible professional life.

2. *Patient characteristics.* Many practitioners prefer to treat young, neurotically ill individuals whom they believe respond best to their psychotherapeutic modalities. Certainly these patients are more pleasant to treat, because they tend to be more similar to ourselves. The Joint Commission on Mental Illness and Health (1961), however, pointed out forcefully that the major unfinished business of psychiatry in America is to provide treatment services for individuals experiencing a major psychiatric illness.

Caregivers in any American community, if queried, indicate that they need help from psychiatric specialists in dealing with individuals who are experiencing failure in some central life role. They will also request assistance with individuals who trouble or concern others in the community by their behavior, in addition to experiencing some failure in adequacy of instrumental functioning. The community will invariably request that the center direct its attention to individuals experiencing major psychoses, to individuals who are socially disabled, and to behavior and personality problems. In the United States, the mental health professional has been most loath to invest his efforts in these individuals. The extent to which the comprehensive community mental health center does deploy its resources in dealing with major psychiatric morbidity and social inadequacy determines its effectiveness as a public mental health program.

3. *Services offered.* If the center offers only psychotherapy, for example, it will be of relatively limited usefulness for the kind of patients that have been discussed in the preceding section. On the other hand, if the only service offered were pharmacotherapy, it would be of very little benefit to the character and behavior problems which concern community caregivers. To some extent, the National Institute of Mental Health has defined the services by listing the five essential and five desirable services. Even within that broad outline, however, there is a wide range of variation. Outpatient services, for example, range all the way from a medication program to a group therapy program to an individual psychotherapy program. It is the conviction of this author that the outpatient program should be eclectic with a vengeance. Also, the full range of offerings of

available psychiatric change technology should exist within the treatment program. Likewise, inpatient service may range all the way from a traditional general hospital psychiatric ward ("a doctor's workshop") to a therapeutic milieu utilizing an extensive sociotherapeutic program. Ideally, the center should probably have available both kinds of inpatient services; some patients are not optimally served by a sociotherapeutic program and would benefit more from the traditional program based on sanctuary, medication, support from personnel, and low demand milieu therapy.

Utilization is a function of patient convenience and perceived patient benefit. Some further discussion is in order concerning utilization, since much of our attention in the early development of comprehensive community mental health centers has gone towards expanding our service clientele. Attempts in most centers to enhance patient convenience include the following:

1. *Decentralization.* Increasingly, mental health centers deploy small groups of staff in neighborhood-based mental health facilities so that they are readily available to patients. This not only increases geographic and temporal availability, but also reduces the cost of utilization of the service as well as significantly reducing the stigmatization. Patients going to a store-front clinic or to a clinic housed in a residential neighborhood find it more convenient, more pleasant, and less frightening than going to a large medical center or psychiatric facility.

2. *Immediate appointments.* Also, mental health facilities are deploying staff to allow a walk-in

capability at the neighborhood level, so that the patient experiencing a crisis need not even wait for an initial appointment but simply appears at the clinic.

3. *Minimizing intake and other administrative procedures.* Centers are moving towards the private practice model by insuring that the initial contact the patient has is with the primary clinician who will assume responsibility for his treatment. Securing admission details and necessary demographic and other information is delayed until it does not interfere with the patient's motivation to utilize service.

4. *Other facilitating efforts.* These include baby-sitting, a nursery for children, free transportation, and home treatment services.

Perceived patient benefit is influenced, of course, by the convenience factor. If the patient is seen immediately upon experiencing severe distress, his perception of benefit will be increased. We know that if patients are not seen at the moment of crisis, most of them will feel somewhat less uncomfortable in a few days; in the past, we have used this to rationalize our delaying practices. It is to our advantage, however, to try to establish a relationship with the patient without delay, knowing he will almost certainly feel better soon and will ascribe some of the benefit to the therapeutic transaction.

There has also been confusion about the utilization of psychotropic medication. A nonsensical extension of psychoanalytic theory claims that since anxiety is a necessary motivating force for psychotherapy, the patient should be left as anxious as possible so motivation will remain high. This implies that the patient is either very stupid or is a masochist, since it is not good judgment to continue to seek help from a practitioner who is not able to offer significant relief of symptoms. A recent study by the author and others (1969) has demonstrated that for an unselected outpatient population experiencing anxiety, the administration of a psychoactive drug—as compared with double-blind administration of placebo—results in a higher rate of perseverance in outpatient treatment and a higher rate of acceptance of definitive therapy recommendations. Individuals are more likely to continue a relationship which results in dramatic relief from symptoms. Patients are also more likely to have confidence in the practitioner who brings about such relief and follow his recommendations for continuing psychotherapeutic assistance. This seems quite reasonable from a common-sense point of view, but strangely enough it has been a controversial point in American psychiatric practice.

The deployment of treatment response appropriate to the severity of discomfort and/or disability of the patient is an important dimension of increasing perceived patient benefit. Rather than being locked into a "one-hour-a-week" structure, a community mental health practitioner should be prepared to deploy clinical resources appropriate to the situation at hand. This may require daily sessions personally with the patient; it may require the utilization of the telephone for frequent telephone contacts; it may require the assignment of a Visiting Nurse or a neighborhood aide for home visits; or it may require the marshalling of massive situational support utilizing the family and also such public agencies as Homemakers. The important thing is that the patient perceives that the clinician is concerned about him as a unique individual and is offering everything humanly possible to decrease his discomfort and increase his adequacy. It is precisely this kind of multifaceted response which characterizes the comprehensive community mental health center in contrast to the preexisting traditional systems of psychiatric care.

In summary, the clinician in a comprehensive community mental health center practices in a new social institution, which is experimental to some extent. He is working in a behavior setting that is more complex than any formerly existing psychiatric institution in the United States. He is locked into a conceptual and operational framework which does not allow him as much right of personal and professional privilege as he often enjoyed in other clinical settings. The clinician works in an institution which has a defined social contract with the community it serves, and often with state and national government. He collaborates with a group of professional colleagues who have not only varying degrees of clinical competence, but also varying degrees of understanding of the nature and the function of a comprehensive community mental health center. The clinician will also encounter different understanding of and sympathy with the contract between the center and its constituency. He functions in a setting where he cannot remain isolated and "do his own thing" without undermining the very meaning and purpose of existence of the comprehensive community mental health center. He must work as a member of a multidisciplinary team if the goals of comprehensiveness and continuity of care are to be realized. He must leave his office; he must be willing to have a flexible schedule; he must cope with ambiguity and unpredictability if the goals of availability, convenience, and perceived patient benefit are to be achieved.

Subsequent chapters will attempt to spell out some of the ways in which traditional clinical practice may be adapted to the unique demands and the unparalleled opportunities of community psychiatric practice within the particular context of the comprehensive community mental health center.

CHAPTER II

The Psychiatric Evaluation

THE PSYCHIATRIC EVALUATION serves three functions: to establish rapport with the patient; to develop a rational treatment plan; and to initiate a psychological contract for treatment between the prospective patient and the treator. The complexity of the evaluative process should in general be a function of the number of treatment alternatives available.

In its search for scientific standing, psychiatry has imbued the evaluation process with a number of ritualistic and pseudoscientific characteristics. Most psychiatric evaluation systems (Menninger, 1962) assume that a medical system of history taking and examination, translated into psychiatric practice, is the most functional evaluative approach. On the surface, this concept appears valid. A careful examination of the actual treatment experience of many patients subjected to such an exhaustive and pseudoscientific evaluation, however, reveals little of the data collected is particularly relevant to decisions about treatment career or events occurring during the course of treatment. Many clinicians are of-

15

ten unaware of the irrelevancies of actual content in the evaluation procedure. To them, evaluation *is* important for their sense of security and personal adequacy. The author is not proposing a solipsistic position, that obtaining information about the patient is unimportant; rather, that the evaluation process should be geared to meeting the needs of the patient, not those of the clinician. Hopefully, younger practitioners in the mental health professions will be trained in settings in which their sense of personal adequacy will not depend so heavily upon aping their colleagues in the physical and biological sciences. If they are strongly rooted in the humanistic tradition, they may be more receptive to the complex transactional qualities of the evaluation process.

Establishing rapport with the patient is a much-discussed, little-understood phenomenon. The patient always comes with certain secret doubts: Will he reject me because I am bad? Will he laugh at me? Will he understand? Is he really competent to help? Will he allow me to behave as outrageously towards him as I have towards other people in my life? Will he hurt me? By his own verbal and non-verbal responses, the clinician must answer each of these questions as they emerge through direct or metaphorical verbalizations and/or through behavior. Such deep concerns, which determine whether the patient and the prospective clinician will even have a relationship, are seldom directly expressed by patients. Rather, they are conveyed metaphorically, by commenting, "If my father heard what I'm telling you, he would be very angry and probably kick me out of the house," to which the therapist may respond, "I suppose you are concerned that I might be angry at you, also." They are also conveyed by behavior such as being late or missing an appointment. In this way, the patient poses the question, "Does he really want to see me? Will he let me get by with manipulating him and behaving in such an outrageous fashion? Will he become angry at me and reject me?"

There is a series of steps that most patients and clinicians go through in the process of establishing rapport. First is the encounter. Our rules used to be beguilingly easy, but fortunately for the welfare of patients, they have become much less simplistic. We took it for granted that the patient was suffering, and wanted help. He had to be willing to wait until it was convenient for us to see him, conforming to our time schedule. The patient then came to our office at an appointed time and stayed for a designated number of minutes. What we developed, in other words, was a belief system and strategy well suited to the needs of moral masochists, who in this country have characteristically made up the bulk of private psychiatric patients. The willingness to submit and suffer in order to obtain psychiatric treatment became only another pathological event in a lifetime of such distorted interpersonal transactions.

In community psychiatry, increasing emphasis must be placed upon the willingness of the therapist to accommodate himself to the needs of the patient. Since each of us has a specific number of hours during a week, a limited supply of energy, and many other commitments to self, family and community, this emphasis stresses our personal and professional resources and our ingenuity. Multidisciplinary team practice seems to be the most workable way to assure constant readiness of response to the needs of patients, while maintaining necessary privacy and autonomy on the part of the individual clinician. When a patient hurts, he hurts now. When he wants help, he wants help now. When he feels bad, he wants to feel better soon, as he would if he went to a physician. When he does not know what to do and is confused, he desires clarity and direction from the clinician. When he has lost his freedom because of overcertainty and overcontrol, he needs openness and permissiveness from the clinician. These needs must all be responded to in the initial encounter.

The initial few minutes of the interview strongly influence its course and productivity and that of the subsequent interviews (Jacobson and Whittington, 1960). Many clinicians have been trained, by example if not by words, to believe the safest route to pursue with all patients is one of cold aloofness, which is a travesty on professionalism. The assumption is that the patient will somehow be put off, offended, or frightened by the human qualities of the individual practitioner. This behavior is terribly dysfunctional in the entire treatment process, since our task with many patients is to help them learn greater self-acceptance and achieve greater comfort with their humanness, with their distinct and often immutable characteristics as unique individuals. A machine-like therapist cannot help the patient achieve these goals. It is true that warmth and genuineness cannot be taught in a training program; it is also unfortunately true, however, that many clinicians have been taught to conceal their warmth and genuineness behind a pseudoscientific facade. A clinician who can say to the patient by his behavior, "I am not ashamed of who I am, nor afraid to be human; perhaps I can help you become less afraid?", is tremendously helpful to his patients.

Next in the evaluation process, the patient must present the "ticket of admission." Virginal psychiatric patients rarely present an entirely appropriate ticket of admission. While few people any longer are naive enough to come in to "ask about a friend," a variety of spurious and irrelevant reasons for seeking help are often presented. It is extremely important that the evaluator not accept an invalid ticket, since beginning the evaluation on an erroneous assumption will distort the process and endanger the development of a workable treatment contract.

In community psychiatric practice, most clinicians begin to focus very quickly on the immediate life context which precipitated the approach to the center. After hearing the initial formulation of the problem by the patient, which is often accompanied by a great deal of intellectual "psychologizing" about the genetic antecedents of the present difficulty, the clinician says something like, "I can understand how concerned you must have been about yourself over the years, since it sounds to me like you have been very uncomfortable and haven't really been able to make out of your life what you had hoped you could. But, I wonder if we could focus a little bit upon how you decided to come see me today. Why didn't you come a month ago or two years ago, or next week or a year from now? I wonder if there wasn't some straw that broke the camel's back, that led you to the decision to come here." An attempt is made, then, to place the patient's symptoms and intrapsychic events within the matrix of current reality and his interpersonal nexus.

Refocusing on the immediate occurrences precipitating a request for psychiatric help is useful in defining the patient's reality situation and in directing his attention upon intrapsychic events and interpersonal and situational variables. It also helps the therapist to develop a rational treatment plan, distinguishing between reinstitution of the premorbid level of functioning and more ambitious treatment goals for modification of the preillness personality pathology.

This process can take from a few minutes to many hours, depending upon the characteristics of the patient and the skill of the clinician. When the therapist is convinced the patient has presented a reasonable "ticket of admission," he must indicate so by verbal and/or behavioral means. The clinician may say something like, "I can understand how you decided to come see me; you have been very tense lately and found yourself unable to overcome the fears you've told me about. What we need to do now is talk some more about the development of these symptoms and a little bit about what kind of person you are and how you came to be that kind of person. The purpose of all of this is so that I can understand what might be most useful to you at this time."

In effect, then, the clinician has legitimized the presenting complaints of the patient. He has said that he should indeed have access to a treatment career, and that a mental health professional is the appropriate person to provide this treatment. He is not at this point giving the patient access to a patient role in which there is any limitation of personal responsibility or lessening of social expectations. Empathy is the penicillin of psychiatry. The clinician's most valuable tool in establishing rapport with the patient is his use of empathic communications. There is ample evidence that a patient's pain and despair can be reduced, his sense of isolation decreased, and self-acceptance increased by the use of only empathic communications. The best rule for the inexperienced clinician is: When in doubt, empathize. If tempted to confront the patient, try to recast the same communication in an empathic fashion. When tempted to interpret, in a genetic or psychodynamic sense, consider the substitution of empathy or precede the interpretation with an empathic comment.

For example, a patient has told a therapist about a long series of struggles with authority. The string of encounters goes back to his father and seems to have involved every significant adult in an authority position in school, college, the military, and at work. The clinician has several choices:

1. He may say nothing.
2. He may confront the patient by saying, "It sounds to me like you fight with everybody who is in a position of authority."
3. He may interpret and say, "It sounds to me as

though you keep acting out your anger towards your father with every person you run into who is in a position of potential authority towards you."

4. Or he may do the same thing empathically by saying, "You must have found it very discouraging to have so many relationships with important people in your life end up badly." The therapist may subsequently say, "I am sure in addition to being discouraged about this, you must have puzzled over how this has happened with you."

The purposes of any of these communications would be the same: to encourage the patient to more realistically observe his own behavior; to make connections between the genetic past and present interpersonal and intrapsychic events; and to facilitate the free flow of communication, affording both the patient and therapist further insight into understanding the maladaptive behavior. I believe the last goal—facilitating communication—is most often achieved by an empathic communication without sacrificing the goals of self-awareness, understanding the relationship of the genetic antecedents, or ability to modify behavior.

Important in developing rapport is the clinician's role as an expert. Many mental health practitioners have found this a difficult task to undertake, wedded as they are to an egalitarian myth system. The patient is not paid for the time that he spends with us, and we are paid. Any logical man would assume this is because the practitioner has a service or a product that is of value, that he is an expert. The reluctance of so many mental health practitioners to display certificates, diplomas, and licenses on their walls is at best an amusing idiosyncrasy of our profession and at worse, a major inconvenience to the patient. The patient wants, and has the right, to know the location, duration, and type of our professional training. He has a right to know licensure and certification status, to know how long we have been in practice, and the exact dimensions of our experience. The clinician who refuses to deal with such issues by open communication when such questions are posed has substantially vitiated his usefulness to the patient. We are not practitioners of an occult art: Our claims to professional competence should not be hidden.

The patient needs to hear whether the practitioner believes that he can be of help with the particular kind of problem posed. In my opinion, this communication should be made clearly and unequivocally during the evaluation process. It is an important part of the solidification of rapport between patient and clinician. The practitioner may say, "While everybody's different and I don't pretend to really understand as much as I need to about you, from the short time that we have talked I think I can tell you that symptoms such as yours usually respond to psychiatric treatment quite well. I am convinced we can work out a treatment plan that will be practical and useful to you."

THE DEVELOPMENT OF A RATIONAL TREATMENT PLAN

Once rapport has been established, the clinician elicits the data necessary to develop a rational treat-

ment plan by utilizing the associative anamnesis
method of interviewing. The clinician should only
obtain information relevant to the decision-making
process he must go through. The general principle
mentioned in the first page of this chapter should be
reiterated: The complexity of the data collection
portion of the evaluation should be a function of the
number of treatment alternatives available within
the setting.

Most practitioners must answer a number of questions for themselves before they can decide which of
the psychiatric change technologies are most appropriate for a particular patient. First, the clinician
needs to know *how* the patient is psychosocially disabled. And second, he needs to know *how severe* is
the psychosocial decompensation. A number of judgments are involved in making this estimation.

1. *Subjective discomfort and distress.* This is an
important variable which must be appraised from
the mass of verbal and nonverbal data collected by
the therapist in his face-to-face encounters with the
patient. One cannot only rely upon the verbal statement, "I'm miserable," but must also supplement
this with behavioral observations. Subjective discomfort is obviously difficult to estimate, and the
therapist's own life style will undoubtedly influence
some of his discriminations about an individual's
degree of discomfort. Experienced clinicians can, however, achieve considerable agreement in rating a patient on a one-to-seven rating scale with the points
being: 1—none, 2—mild/intermittent, 3—mild/con-
tinued, 4—moderate/intermittent, 5—severe/inter-
mittent, 6—moderate/continual, 7—severe/continual.

There are a handful of patients, however, who tend to polarize staff opinion. Certain staff members see them as experiencing severe subjective discomfort, while others see them as callous, manipulative and theatrical. These patients are most often women, characteristically from family environments marked by severe parental conflict in which they played a pivotal role. Not infrequently, over a period of time they develop behaviors that come eventually to be labeled psychotic or schizophrenic.

2. *The patient's effect on his environment.* The actual effect achieves inter-rater agreement relatively easily while the potential effect is more subject to individual interpretation. Again, most patients can be rated on a continuum between no discomfort inflicted to destruction of person and/ or property, in physical and/or emotional terms.

3. *Seriousness of the symptoms.* This is a complex judgment that requires balancing a number of dimensions of personality functioning. Judgments tend to be based upon our normative expectations of age-appropriate behavior. We expect people in our society to have a number of characteristics:

a. First, we expect them to be able to tell between external reality and internal fantasies the majority of the time.

b. We expect their perception of sensory input from the environment to conform rather closely to that of other individuals in the same environment.

c. We expect them to be able to utilize logical thought processes to solve problems and to adapt to the demands of the environment.

d. We expect them to respond in emotionally understandable ways, which seem appropriate or related to the stimulus causing the emotion.

e. We expect them to be able to delay impulses for a reasonable period of time, postponing the gratification of such impulses until their expression is congruent with environmental, interpersonal, and intrapsychic factors.

f. We expect adults to have a well-developed sense of judgment to anticipate the consequences of various behaviors so they are able to avoid maladaptive responses to environmental pressures.

g. We expect individuals not to harm themselves through self-destructive behavior in either a symbolic, displaced, or direct form.

It should be emphasized that subjective discomfort and seriousness of symptoms are not related in a linear fashion. There is a general correlation between them, but individual patients may show wide variations between these two dimensions.

4. *Dependence upon situational support and vulnerability to situational stress.* These may be evaluated from the patient's history and also within the clinical setting. Proceeding with the associative anamnesis, the community psychiatric practitioner tries to obtain full understanding of prior periods of psychosocial decompensation. He is trying to understand the severity and duration of the situational stresses and the exact quality of the situational supports, either present or lacking. These concerns are in addition to the traditional psychiatric interest in the intrapsychic meaning of the particular stress.

The patient's response to stress may be evaluated

within the clinical situation. The hospital or day hospital setting is an excellent opportunity to understand more about the patient's vulnerability to external pressures. It is also possible to stress the patient, in the individual evaluation interview, at least for short periods of time. This should be done, however, only after rapport is well established and the clinician has considerable confidence in his ability to maintain a relationship with the patient. Silence is almost universally stressful to patients, as is withholding empathic comments after establishing a pattern of empathic communication. Withholding affective or nonverbal behavioral cues by the therapist is stressful; challenging and confronting behavior by the therapist also may be utilized. None of these techniques should be resorted to unless there is a specific question that needs to be answered as a necessary part of developing a rational treatment plan. It is not necessary in the evaluation process to reveal the full depth and floridity of the patient's psychopathology: It is not in the best interest of the patient's self-esteem, the therapeutic relationship, or the probability of success in treatment.

If the clinician is wondering whether the patient can tolerate outpatient psychotherapy in his present environmental situation, however, and is uncertain about the answer, he must have some information concerning the patient's stress vulnerability and his dependence upon situational support. If silence and/or the withdrawal of empathic communication and/or confrontation and/or the withdrawal of all responsive behavior on the part of the clinician results in a manifest worsening of the patient's psychosocial capability, thought must be given in the treatment plan to minimizing situational stresses and maximizing situational supports. This may include consideration of hospital or day hospital treatment.

If, on the other hand, the patient responds by counterpressure on the therapist or anger, without any apparent worsening in cognitive processes, impulse control, perception of reality, or judgment, the therapist may conclude that the individual is not overly dependent on situational supports and has a store of ego reserves that give him some resistance to stress. In such a situation, the initial decision may be to formulate an outpatient treatment plan, with some sense of confidence that the patient has the capacity to utilize such a low-support type of treatment career.

5. *The quality of the interpersonal relationships.* This may, again, be evaluated through history and through behavioral observations within the clinical setting. During the evaluation of the patient's interpersonal relationships, a collateral informant may be particularly valuable. Even without this, careful psychiatric interviewing usually gives a fairly accurate profile of the quantitative and qualitative aspects of the interpersonal life of the patient. Again, we are, in effect, judging the patient against certain normative expectations of what we consider "healthy interpersonal behavior" within the context of our particular culture:

a. We expect healthy interpersonal relationships

to have a quality of mutuality. At the other end of the spectrum, we would consider exploitative relationships, in which one individual exploits another to gratify his own needs, as less normative.

b. We expect a significant portion of the interpersonal relationships in an individual's life to be relatively enduring ones. We do not consider it normal in our culture for an individual to only be able to have a relationship for a week or two or for a month, moving through hundreds of individual attachments over a period of years.

c. A certain mixture of love and hate is displayed within any relationship, but we anticipate that enduring relationships will evidence a preponderance of love in the affective repertoire of the individuals involved. We would consider a relationship less "normal" when it is marked by a great deal of ambivalence—by considerable direct or indirect expression of hateful or aggressive strivings.

d. Significant relationships can survive a considerable degree of need frustration. If the relationship is totally dependent upon need gratification, however, and would be terminated at the point the patient's needs are partially frustrated, we would consider it an "unhealthy" relationship.

Individuals who have a high degree of psychosocial adequacy, then, experience many loving and mutual relationships, which are relatively enduring and capable of surviving need frustration. Adaptational casualties, on the other hand, would frequently have interpersonal lives characterized by no meaningful interpersonal relationships or by relationships characterized by impermanence, ambivalence, exploitiveness, and dependency upon need gratification.

6. *Use of abilities.* The degree to which the individual can utilize his abilities must be assessed in determining psychosocial adequacy. One must take into account not only the constitutional anlage of the individual, but also development during crucial childhood years through psychomotor stimulation, education, and cultural opportunities. One must also take into account the individual's access to the opportunity structure within society, recognizing that there are gross disparities based on ethnicity in the United States.

If one saw, then, a southern Negro with an I.Q. of 140 who had not completed high school and was working as a janitor, one would be less inclined to consider the underutilization of his ability as a sign of psychosocial decompensation, than, for example, if one saw the white son of a college professor with an I.Q. of 140 who had a master's degree in psychology working as a janitor. In the first case, the underachievement is likely to be socially determined; in the second case, it is psychologically caused.

7. *The breadth and depth of interests of the individual.* Many persons who are defined as adaptational casualties or labeled as psychiatric patients are extremely impoverished in both the breadth and the depth of their interests. Much of this is due to interpersonal and situational impoverishment during the early years of those who subsequently become psychosocially maladapted.

It is characteristic of some patients with minor degrees of psychosocial impairment to overconcentrate on certain interests at the expense of breadth, becoming superspecialists or zealots in a particular area of human endeavor. Others tend to maintain the interest pattern characteristic of adolescents in our culture, with a great breadth of interest, but no depth because the individual is unable to abandon options, limiting his potential freedom of maneuver in order to invest his energies in certain special interest areas. The psychosocially best adapted people in our society, we would postulate, are those who have a flexible balance between breadth and depth of interests.

8. *The trend of the decompensation.* This is crucial in determining treatment strategy. If the condition seems to be rapidly improving, for example, one tends to consider the psychosocial decompensation less severe, or at least less demanding of professional mental health intervention. To the extent that the psychosocial decompensation is static or rapidly deteriorating, a somewhat more ominous import is indicated.

9. *Chronicity must be appraised.* As a general rule of thumb, a state of impaired psychosocial decompensation that is persistent for two or more years presents treatment and rehabilitation problems which are quite different from less chronic conditions. As subjective discomfort persists, as the patient's effect on his environment continues to be noxious, as the seriousness of his symptoms brings about impairment of his adaptive capacity, as his

dependence upon situational support persists and his vulnerability to situational stress endures, as the quality of his interpersonal relationships remains inadequate, as he is unable to utilize his abilities, as he is impoverished in breadth and depth of interests, and as his condition deteriorates, complex feedback mechanisms from significant others in the patient's immediate environment, as well as from the larger social environment in which he lives, tend to reinforce the pattern of psychosocial decompensation and to erode the individual's sense of personal self-worth and adequacy. He comes increasingly to "burn his psychological and interpersonal bridges behind him." A treatment plan for such a chronically ill patient, then, cannot simply focus upon the removal of symptoms. It must also give consideration to planning for social relearning through guided group interaction. In many instances, it must provide for the learning or relearning of social adaptational skills of other sorts, including instrumental functioning related to the role expectations imposed on the individual within his family and within society.

The community mental health practitioner must remember that chronicity and institutionalism do not occur only within state hospitals. People may become just as chronically disabled for successful interpersonal adjustment and role competence while living in their own homes and while being treated in a comprehensive community mental health center, as they did in the snakepits of yesteryear. The same feedback mechanisms and reinforcement of maladaptive, sick role behavior which occur in state hos-

pitals, and which have been so brilliantly documented, can and do occur equally in other settings.

In a community mental health setting, if the
judgment of the clinician after answering the above
listed questions is that the patient is only mildly
decompensated psychosocially, and that there is
some evidence of reconstitution, the clinician may
decide to defer treatment for several months in order to evaluate the potential for spontaneous cure.
We all know that each of us experiences periods of
psychosocial decompensation under a variety of internal and external events, and that in the vast
majority of instances reconstitutive efforts on the
part of the individual within his immediate and social milieu are successful in returning him to a premorbid level of functioning. Since the community
mental health center never has adequate treatment
resources, relative to demand, it is particularly important that discriminating judgments be made to
defer treatment of individuals where there is reasonable expectation of spontaneous cure. In such cases,
the individual may be told, "As we have talked
these last few hours, I think it has become pretty
clear what's been happening to you, and I think we
both know a lot of reasons why you've been so upset
lately. Everything that we've talked about so far,
however, indicates that you had already begun to
make progress in coping with these problems before
you came to see me, and this progress seems to be
continuing. You've handled difficulties like this in
the past, and I think we have every reason to expect
that you will continue to work this out without any
further psychiatric treatment at the present time. I

would suggest that we go on that assumption for the next three months, and set up an appointment to get together then to make sure that everything is going okay and to reevaluate the situation."

In community psychiatric practice, there are some situations in which this option of no treatment in the hope of spontaneous cure will not be exercised:

1. If it is crucial for the individual to maintain optimal coping effectiveness—a mother with young children or a husband with a psychiatrically or physically ill wife with young children—the decision may be made to institute treatment as the better part of valor.

2. If community concern is very great about the individual either because the patient's effect upon others is noxious or because his condition represents significant slippage from a position of extraordinary competence and responsibility, making his psychosocial decompensation seem more ominous than it may really be, then it might be desirable to offer treatment immediately.

3. If the immediate family and/or community caregivers ("pseudofamily") are openly hostile to the patient and are utilizing destructive behaviors, it may be wise to offer therapeutic intervention promptly.

When an individual is severely decompensated in his psychosocial adequacy, in the presence of fixed resources and limited change technology, the community mental health practitioner must still decide whether he should invest treatment resources; and if so, how intensive and how prolonged the investment should be. In order to make this judgment, some indication of the prognosis for the individual involved should be investigated, since in general, a clinician will tend to invest his resources in cases with a prognosis that is not poor.

Again, the estimation of prognosis involves a multifactorial judgment, based upon the clinical experience of the practitioner who utilizes data derived from the interview, collateral history, and behavioral observations.

1. Premorbid adjustment is probably the most sensitive and valid predictor of therapeutic potential. It requires no great scientific sophistication to arrive at this decision, since most of us operate with the probability estimate that the best predictor of future behavior is past behavior. We should not discard this common-sense rule of thumb in our role as mental health practitioner.

2. Again, the duration of symptoms is extremely important in determining the patient's treatment potential. If severe symptoms persist for longer than two years, most evidence indicates that prognosis begins to worsen rapidly after that period of time.

3. We tend to believe that individuals experiencing a serious psychosocial decompensation as a consequence of a severe prolonged stress or catastrophic precipitating event, have a generally better treatment prognosis than those who become adaptational casualties in the presence of slight or no known situational stresses.

4. Although theoretical formulations of the reasons are inexact, most clinicians believe the retention of affective responsivity on the part of the patient is a good prognostic indicator. Bland or flat affect, severe inhibition in the range and intensity of

affect, and/or inappropriate and/or unmodulated affectivity, on the other hand, tend to suggest a less favorable prognosis.

5. Motivation for change, however, has been over-utilized as a prognostic indicator. There is certainly evidence that patients treated under coercion—as are many patients who are involuntarily committed to psychiatric hospitals—can benefit materially from therapeutic intervention. To the extent that treatment is prolonged, is weighted heavily towards psychoanalytically-oriented psychotherapy, requires activity and commitment on the part of the patient, and produces uncomfortable reactions, motivation becomes a more crucial variable. Again, the clinician should be alert not only to verbal expressions of motivation, but also to behavioral indications. The patient who protests against therapy and will have none of it, but who comes on time to his appointments regularly, is obviously much more motivated than the patient who verbally expresses his great faith in and commitment to treatment, but who characteristically is late for or misses appointments.

6. Ego strength is another important prognostic indicator. Unfortunately, consensus between raters about ego strength in an individual tends to be disparate. Ego strength may be defined as the extent and adequacy of the adaptive repertoire of the individual. If he has faced and coped with major life stresses and adaptational demands, we have evidence that his ego strength is considerable. If he has characteristically failed to rise to such adaptational demands, we would estimate that his ego strength is low. If there is impoverishment in his repertoire of

adaptive capacities—a fixed response to stress such as always drinking, always running away, or always developing somatic complaints—we would delineate his ego strength or adaptive capacity as low. When a person evidences a wide range of adaptational capability—so that at various times he might have gotten drunk to escape, fought to discharge aggression, found another job to increase his financial resources to cope with environmental demands, attended school to increase his adaptive repertoire—we describe his ego strength as great.

The estimation of ego strength becomes increasingly difficult in our society, as more and more people are raised in the age of affluence without major adaptive demands placed upon them. The author cannot say that a lifetime of indulgence and predictability produces people who have poor ego strength; but he can say that it makes it extremely difficult, in evaluating a patient, to know what his ability to respond to stress is when he has been exposed to very few stresses beyond the range of the ordinary and anticipated ones in the course of his life.

7. Psychological-mindedness has been considered an extremely important variable for psychotherapeutically-oriented treatment careers. Evidence of successful psychotherapy with lower socioeconomic individuals, who have been reported not to be psychology-minded, and with mentally retarded individuals, suggests that we have been overdependent on this variable as a prognostic indicator.

8. Likeableness of the patient, while difficult to quantify, is clearly important in estimating prognosis.

This statement is based on the assumption that while the patient is in treatment, he also lives in a real world populated by other people. When his behavior is repulsive and offensive, he evokes rejection, anger, disparagement, ridicule, and punishment. When he is "likeable," as defined by the folk-hero and myth systems of the particular culture, he is likely to elicit approbation, reward, assistance, encouragement, love, and appreciation. The partial meeting of psychological needs through extratherapeutic encounters not only makes therapy easier, but also allows a more predictable return to psychosocial adequacy.

9. Faith in therapy tends to be weighted very highly by many psychotherapeutic practitioners. By itself it is valueless as a prognostic indicator. Faith in therapy does have some importance, however, when it is offered psychotherapeutically and requires the patient's acceptance of the therapist's belief system about the motivation of human behavior and the adoption of a new value system.

10. Externalization has been viewed as an ominous prognostic indicator for therapeutic intervention. Most therapists experience great difficulty in engaging themselves with patients who see problems as entirely outside themselves and find it relatively easy to treat patients who see all problems as internal. In other words, we have characteristically found it easier to deal with moral masochists than with activists. Although we included externalization in the prognostic schema—as we did faith in therapy, psychological-mindedness, and motivation for change—we are not commenting upon any inherent

prediction of prognosis related to these characteristics. We are rather talking about the characteristic fate of individuals in the American system, being treated by mental health practitioners as currently trained, and operating with the myth, belief, and preference system that influences most mental health practitioners at the present time.

In the community mental health setting, if the overall prognosis is considered poor, the decision to afford treatment would be dependent upon whether the offering of treatment would deprive other individuals with a better prognosis of all access to a treatment career. If so, treatment within the community mental health setting would not be offered. An attempt would be made to marshal situational supports utilizing nonpsychiatric caregiving professionals and agencies within the community.

The clinician must also decide whether he will recommend hospitalization or whether he will attempt to treat the individual as an outpatient if the psychosocial decompensation is very great. In doing this, he asks himself the following questions: (a) Is there evidence of active suicidal preoccupation in the fantasy or thoughts of the patient? (In arriving at this decision, a suicidal potential scale may be utilized.) (b) Have there been recent suicidal attempts or active preparation to harm himself (i.e., buying a gun, etc.)? (c) Has the patient threatened to hurt someone else physically? (d) Have aggressive outbursts occurred towards people? (e) Have aggressive outbursts occurred towards animals? Objects? (f) Has antisocial behavior of other sorts occurred? (g) Are there evidences of impairment of such functions as reality assessment, judgment, logical thinking, and planning? (h) Does the patient's condition seem to be deteriorating rapidly despite supportive measures? (i) Are there physical or neurological conditions which require hospital rehabilitation services? (j) Do pathological social or family situations exist that require isolation of the patient? (k) Are the emotional contacts of the patient so severely limited that the "push" of a structured hospital program may be helpful?

Again, this multifactorial judgment will, at best, give the clinician some rough guidelines in deciding whether to recommend hospital or outpatient treatment. The day hospital allows the clinician more flexibility in arriving at this decision. A period of day hospitalization may help clarify the patient's need for hospitalization or ability to utilize outpatient treatment.

A rating scale that has been used experimentally for estimating psychosocial decompensation and for determining a rational treatment plan is included for the interest of readers. Please be reminded, however, that this is not a standardized or validated clinical instrument, but simply is in experimental usage in our center at the present time.

THE TREATMENT CONTRACT

Once the clinician has completed the evaluation process and has gathered and synthesized the data available to him, it is incumbent upon him to make a clear presentation of his findings to the patient

and/or the family. He must also make recommendations. In doing this, he should discuss the following
topics:

1. *How is the patient psychosocially maladapted?*
The symptoms and signs of psychosocial decompensation should be described in nontechnical language
to the extent that the clinician believes the patient
and/or the family can use this as a legitimation of
the need for psychiatric treatment.

2. *How psychosocially decompensated is the
patient?* A clear statement of severity should be
offered. Equivocation or evasion of the issues of severity or chronicity rarely is in the best interest of
the patient or significant others in his life. While we
do not want to label people schizophrenic or hopeless and incurable, we do need to clearly describe—
unless there is compelling evidence to the contrary
—the severity of the problem. The clinican may want
to say what he thinks will happen if treatment is not
undertaken if the patient and/or the family should
be resistant to the recommendation for a specific
therapeutic intervention.

3. *Why is the individual psychosocially maladapted?* Most psychiatric practitioners in the
United States today are preoccupied with this question. The bulk of their professional time is spent
eliciting information related to the psychogenetic
antecedents of particular personality traits and maladaptive behaviors and constructing cause and effect
fantasies about prior interpersonal and intrapsychic
events and present behavior. This is rarely useful to

a patient and/or family at the initiation of treatment, though it is entertaining and of some use for many mental health practitioners.

If the present symptomatology is related to noxious or conflicted interpersonal relationships in the current life space of the patient, and/or to other situational stresses, however, the information may have great relevance for the patient and/or his family. For example, it makes great sense to a patient to say, "I think you're having diarrhea all the time because of the trouble that's going on between you and your wife." It is not at all useful to patients to say, "I think the diarrhea you're having all the time is because of the way your mother toilet trained you." In speaking about the why of the patient's symptoms, the clinician is also reinforcing a part of the rapport, in terms of establishing his status as an expert who can and will help the patient.

4. *What treatment is recommended?* A full discussion should be made here of the type, frequency, duration, expense, and probable outcome of the treatment process. While we cannot predict with any high degree of exactitude how many weeks or months the patient may be in treatment, we really have some very good estimates from our prior treatment experiences. If the patient wants this information, some time estimate should be given. If we attempt to evade such questions, we are simply eroding the patient's sense that we are indeed expert and know what we are doing; we also dilute his trust in our candor and our ability to share our special knowledge.

Nothing will be gained by putting an unjustifiably optimistic cast on the likely outcome of treatment. Many patients know how dreadfully ill they are; our attempts to be overly optimistic simply vitiate our credibility. During therapy, a patient is never lost by telling him he is a complicated person and his illness is very difficult to treat, and you will stick with him through the treatment process. Many a patient is lost by being told that his illness is not serious and shouldn't take long to get straightened out—when he knows perfectly well that is not true.

Telling the partners in a hopelessly bitter marriage that marriage counseling, group therapy, or individual psychotherapy for one or both of them will make everything all right is pointless. No form of psychiatric treatment can erase the past, and despite our most Pollyannaish wishes, no psychiatric treatment can repair a human relationship eroded by years of bitterness and mutual infliction of pain.

Psychiatric evaluation methods can only be learned through the preceptor method, by actually working with patients with the assistance of a more experienced colleague. The opportunity to repeatedly observe others who are more experienced is an important addition in learning to conduct evaluations. Reporting all transactions to a supervisor, having one's interviews observed directly through closed-circuit television and commented upon by a teaching colleague, and observing one's own interviews on video-tape are factors which are important in learning to conduct competent psychiatric evaluations.

PSYCHIATRIC PATIENT DATA FORM

PATIENT'S NAME: _____ AGE: ___ SEX: ___ DATE: ___

Descriptive Diagnosis: _____

Score _____

Rating Scale For Estimating Psychosocial Decompensation

1. The patient's *subjective discomfort and distress:*

1	2	3	4	5	6	7
Severe, Continual	Moderate, Continual	Severe, Intermittent	Moderate, Intermittent	Mild, Continual	Mild, Intermittent	None

2. The patient's *effect on his environment* (actual or potential):

1	2	3	4	5	6	7
Very destructive of person and property			Inflicts moderate discomfort			No discomfort inflicted

3. *The seriousness of the symptoms:*

1	2	3	4	5	6	7
Gross distortion of reality: autistic regression	Some disturbance of perceptual clarity	Disruption of cognitive & affective functioning	Isolated defects in cognitive & affective functioning	Appraisal of reality relatively intact, except during periods of severe anxiety	Occasional symptoms	No symptoms

Impairment of Impulse Control →

Impairment of Judgment →

Self-Harm →

4. *Dependence on Situational Support* (and vulnerability to situational stress):

1	2	3	4	5	6	7
Totally Dependent	Can function only with massive external support	Very vulnerable to stress	With some support can tolerate most stress	A little "tougher" & "more independent" than most	With minimal support can tolerate severe stress	Extremely resistant to situational stress; independent, autonomous functioning

SCORE

5. The quality of his *interpersonal relationships*:

1	2	3	4	5	6	7
No meaningful interpersonal relationships	Few interpersonal relationships	Marked ambivalence in relationships	Many relationships of "normal" ambivalence	Better than average ability to establish and maintain relationships	"Post-ambivalent"	Many loving and mutual relationships

exploitativeness ———————→ mutual

impermanence ———————→ enduring

dependent upon need–gratification ———————→ survive need–frustration

SCORE _____

6. The degree to which he can *utilize his abilities*:

1	2	3	4	5	6	7
No Utilization			Moderate Utilization			Full Utilization

7. The *breadth and depth of his interests:*

1	2	3	4	5	6	7
Impoverished			Tends to over-concentrate on certain interests at expense of breadth; or *vice versa*			Flexible balance between depth and breadth

8. The *trend* of the decompensation:

1	2	3	4	5	6	7
Static, regressed	Rapidly Deteriorating	Slowly Deteriorating	Stable	Slowly Improving	Rapidly Improving	Evanescent

9. *Chronicity* of the psychosocial decompensation:

1	2	3	4	5	6	7
4 yrs.	3–4 yrs.	2–3 yrs.	1–2 yrs.	6–12 mos.	3–6 mos.	3 mos.

TOTAL SCORE _____

Range	Severity
45–63	"Normal"–Mildly Decompensated
30–44	Mildly–Moderately Decompensated
Under 30	Moderately–Severely Decompensated

If score is 45 or over, defer treatment for three months to evaluate spontaneous care potential *unless*

YES	NO	
___	___	Crucialness of maintaining optimal coping effectiveness is very great; as, mother with young (under five years) child/children; or, husband with psychiatrically or physically ill wife and young children.
___	___	Community concern is very great, either about patient's effect on others or because of his slippage from a position of extraordinary competence and responsibility.
___	___	Relatives and/or caregivers ("pseudofamily") are openly hostile toward patient and demanding therapeutic intervention.

If score is less than 44, determine treatment plan based on available resources, characteristics of the patient, and prognosis (potential yield on investment of therapeutic effort).

Prognostic Schema

Item	Rating	Score	Comments
1. Premorbid Adjustment	1. Very poor		
	2. Poor		
	3. Average		
	4. Good		
	5. ...		

2. Duration of Symptoms	1. More than 3 years 2. 2–3 years 3. 1–2 years 4. 3–12 months 5. Less than 3 months
3. Precipitating Event	1. No known situational stress 2. Slight stress 3. Moderate stress 4. Severe, brief stress 5. Severe, prolonged stress
4. Affect	1. Bland 2. Flat 3. Inhibited range and intensity of affectivity and/or inappropriate and/or unmodulated affectivity 4. Full range of affect but quantitatively inhibited 5. Free affective reactions to psychic conflict and inter-personal events
5. Motivation for Change	1. None 2. Minimal 3. Moderate 4. Very good 5. Great

Item	Rating	Score	Comments
6. "Ego Strength"	1. Minimal 2. Moderate 3. Average 4. Good 5. Great		
7. Psychological-Mindedness	1. None 2. Minimal 3. Average 4. Good 5. Great		
8. "Likableness"	1. Repulsive 2. Irritating 3. Likable 4. Very Likable 5. Charming		
9. "Faith in Therapy"	1. Open scorn or rejection of need 2. Covert scorn or rejection of need 3. Doubting 4. Hopes and believes can help 5. Great Faith		
10. Externalization	1. Sees problems as entirely external 2. Sees problems as largely external 3. Sees problems as partly external 4. Sees most problems as internal 5. Sees all problems as internal		

TOTAL _____

initiating treatment should be seriously examined.

If Psychosocial Decompensation score is less than 30, criteria for hospitalization should be completed as a part of treatment planning.

Criteria For Hospitalization

	Weighting	Score				Weighted Score
		No 0	Slight 1	Moderate 2	Extensive 3	
1. Is there evidence of active suicidal preoccupation, in fantasy or thoughts of patient?*	2					
2. Have there been recent suicidal attempts or active preparation to harm self (i.e., buying gun, etc.)?*	4					
3. Has the patient threatened to hurt someone else physically?	2					
4. Have aggressive outbursts occurred toward animals? Objects?	2					
5. Have aggressive outbursts occurred toward people?	4					
6. Has antisocial behavior occurred?	1					
7. Are there evidences of impairment of such functions as reality assessment, judgment, logical thinking, and planning?	1					
8. Does the patient's condition seem to be deteriorating rapidly despite supportive measures?	1					

	Weighting	Score				Weighted Score
		No 0	Slight 1	Moderate 2	Extensive 3	
9. Are there physical or neurological conditions which require rehabilitation services?	2					
10. Do pathological social or family situations exist that require isolation of the patient?	1					
11. Are emotional contacts of the patient so severely limited that the "push" of a structured hospital program may be helpful?	1					

TOTAL _____

Score of 12 or more: Hospitalization for evaluation mandatory.
Score of 8–11: Outpatient evaluation probably feasible before deciding on hospitalization.
Score of 7 or less: Outpatient treatment probably feasible.

*Suicidal potential scale may be utilized to help in making judgment of suicide risk.

Psychiatric Patient Data Form: Supplement A
Prediction of Suicidal Behavior

                                                    Yes   No   ?

1. Is this person male? ....   —   —   —
2. Is this person Caucasian? ....   —   —   —
3. Is this person 45 years of age or older? ....   —   —   —

5. Does this person live in the transitional area surrounding the central downtown section? . . . . . |

6. Did this person currently attempt suicide by oral ingestion, shooting, or jumping from a high place? . . . . . |

7. Was this person unconscious or unable to answer questions coherently as a result of the self-destructive act? . . . . . |

8. Did this person have a previous psychiatric hospitalization? . . . . . |

9. Did this person make a previous suicide attempt? . . . . . |

10. Was this person in poor physical health during the past 6 months? . . . . . |

11. Does this person now have or has he ever had a problem with alcohol? . . . . . |

12. Does this person now have or has he ever had a problem with drug addiction? . . . . . |

13. Does this person now have or has he ever had a problem with antisocial behavior? . . . . . |

14. Has this person suffered a loss—real, threatened or fantasied—within the past 6 months? . . . . . |

TOTALS ‖ ‖

Instructions for scoring: To obtain a score, total the "yes" answers.

Score Range	Classification	Probability of repeated suicidal behavior within 8 years
0–3	Low Risk	1 in 22
4–6	Moderate Risk	1 in 3
7 or more	Suicide prone	1 in 2

CHAPTER III

Treatment Modalities

THE PURPOSE of treatment may be to promote improvement, to prevent worsening, to slow worsening, and/or to reduce the extent of worsening of a psychiatric illness. In his treatment function, the community mental health practitioner differs significantly from some other mental health practitioners:

1. His stance is always antiregressive. Allowing or promoting regression to more primitive, less adaptive psychosocial functioning is never in the interest of the patient. The emphasis in treatment, therefore, is upon reinforcing and aiding the adaptive capacity of the individual, and/or the family—even if this is at the expense of an associative anamnesis which could result in a better dynamic formulation or at the expense of intellectual insight on the part of the patient or clinician. This characteristic of practice springs from several sources:

a. The never-ending discrepancy between demand for service and available treatment resources propels community mental health practitioners to potentiate the patient's and family's motivation for self-help. We must try to avoid psychosocial regres-

54

sion, which increases personal and social disability, and renders the treatment program more prolonged and difficult.

b. Many community mental health practitioners had their training and early experience in state or Veterans Administration hospitals and in other traditional psychiatric settings. The tendency of such settings to sanction and promote regression, with resultant secondary impairment, impressed many of the leaders in community mental health practice with iatrogenic factors in much psychiatric disability in the United States.

c. Community mental health practitioners have often been surprised at the yield from extremely limited treatment resources extended to individuals who traditionally have been regarded as seriously ill, as needing a quantitatively greater treatment experience. Patients who in other settings would be labeled hopeless or untreatable, often respond to optimistic, vigorous, and pragmatic intervention. Over the years the community mental health practitioner becomes increasingly optimistic about the strength and adaptive capacity of individuals who are labeled as psychiatric patients. Thus he believes with more certainty that people must assume responsibility for their own behavior.

2. The community mental health practitioner is eclectic. In this country, he has most frequently been trained in a setting with an exclusively psychodynamic orientation, often heavily psychoanalytic. His exposure to an unrestricted caseload, if he takes seriously his obligation to the community, quickly leads him to expand the basic dyadic model of psy-

chotherapy and to temper his characteristically American preoccupation with childhood psychogenetic factors.

3. The practitioner in a comprehensive community mental health center has access to many more treatment alternatives than he would have in other settings. He becomes, then, a kind of broker for his patient, not only providing service himself, but also helping the patient obtain needed services within the center.

4. The community mental health practitioner is aware of cost-benefit issues in the provision of treatment services. He lives in a real world where resources have been limited as long as he can remember, and he anticipates that public mental health resources will continue to be less than service demands. As a pragmatic Utopian, he constantly must ask himself whether the investment of treatment resources in a particular patient is warranted by the anticipated yield.

5. The community mental health practitioner is present- and future-oriented. His treatment stance tends to be contemporaneous; his dialogue with the patient phenomenological; his expectation that of improvement.

Not all patients are best served by such an approach. A patient who needed, for example, to enter a psychoanalytic treatment situation, to experience a regressive transference, and to work through his experiences in such a relationship would not be at all well-served by a comprehensive community mental health center. He might be told that he seems to be functioning adequately in his central life roles, that he does not strike the examiner as being any more unhappy than most other people, and that there really seems to be no indication for psychiatric treatment at the present time. If the same patient were to walk into a private psychiatrist's office at the appointed time wearing a suit and tie and had an income of $12,000 a year or better, he would undoubtedly be told that psychotherapy was the treatment choice for his existential dilemma. Who is to say which approach serves the needs of the patient better?

Treatment Options in a Comprehensive Community Mental Health Center

At the end of the psychiatric evaluation, the practitioner in a comprehensive community mental health center should have a wide variety of offerings available.

The Psychotherapies

Psychotherapy may be defined as an encounter between two or more people, of whom at least one is defined as a therapist and at least one is defined as experiencing a psychological or psychiatric illness. Our belief in the efficacy of psychotherapy is based on the following assumptions:

1. It is emotionally relieving to tell another person who is empathic and nonjudgmental, about things which have been troubling one.

2. In this process, the patient may understand certain relationships between his current emotional problems and contemporaneous or past events,

and/or his idiosyncratic emotional responses to those events.

3. The process of psychotherapy may constitute, additionally, a corrective emotional experience, allowing the patient to have a sustained relationship with a predictable and trusted figure who responds to him differently than other significant individuals have in the past.

4. The therapist, by certain of his behaviors, may facilitate a process resulting in changed modes of thinking, feeling, and behaving. The repertoire of therapist behaviors is really quite limited:

a. The therapist may be empathic, indicating his understanding of the patient's reaction to or feeling about a particular internal or external event.

b. The therapist may ask for additional information or clarification, facilitating the process of self-examination on the part of the patient.

c. The therapist may interpret the motivation of a certain behavior or offer interpretive connections between present thoughts, feelings, or behaviors, and antecedent or contemporaneous events causally related to such factors.

d. The therapist may reassure the patient.

e. The therapist may exhort the patient, attempting to mobilize his ego resources in order to increase adaptational capacity.

f. The therapist may instruct the patient, providing him with new information that will be useful to him in coping with his life dilemma.

g. The therapist may confront or challenge the patient, forcefully pointing out to him the exact quality and impact of characteristic ways of behaving.

h. The therapist may reward certain behavior in the therapeutic situation by responding verbally or nonverbally in a pleased or friendly manner; and conversely, may discourage certain other behaviors by negative or noncommittal responses.

There are many ways to classify the psychotherapies. In general, any classification would have to take into account the following factors: the number of people involved; the level of expectation of participants; the degree of control exerted by the therapist; and the theoretical orientation or psychotherapy style of the practitioner.

Dyadic psychotherapy, where the behavioral orientation of the therapist is essentially a modification of psychoanalytic practice, with high expectations of and for the patient and low control of the patient by the therapist, has become over the years the treatment approach taught predominantly in training programs in the United States. This method is judged most efficacious and is viewed as the treatment of highest prestige; and its practice endows the therapist with the highest financial rewards and professional status. It is also the treatment modality with the highest cost per unit of service, whose effectiveness is totally unproven by scientific experimentation. The author is convinced from his own personal experience that individual or dyadic psychotherapy is indeed effective for many patients of all diagnostic categories, ethnic backgrounds, and socioeconomic levels. It is his assumption that most of the individuals reading this book are in the process of developing a similar conviction about the efficacy of psychotherapy, both from their experience as therapists and in many instances from their experience as patients.

The comprehensive community mental health center concept in no way discourages or attempts to supplant or render invalid individual psychodynamically-oriented psychotherapy. Rather, the plea is that this should not be the *only* therapeutic modality in the armamentarium of the community psychiatric practitioner. As a treatment method it should not have higher status (the practitioner higher prestige) than other treatment modalities.

There is some evidence that the theoretical orientation of the practitioner has very little relation to the outcome of psychotherapy; and there is also evidence that it is relatively easy to teach people to be psychotherapists. We have deluded ourselves into thinking that psychotherapy is the most demanding task for the mental health practitioner, mainly because we have developed such an overelaborate ideational system to rationalize our activity or lack of activity as therapists: We end up playing intricate and confusing word games with ourselves and our colleagues. It is quite possible that psychotherapy employed without *any* systematic, theoretically-based interpretation is more effective than psychotherapy which utilizes interpretations rising from a particular theoretical point of view.

It is the conviction of the author that the bulk of routine psychotherapy in the comprehensive community mental health center of the future will be done by individuals trained at the master's degree level or lower.

Group psychotherapy is heavily favored in any comprehensive community mental health center's treatment program. This is partly due to the promise of some economy of effort—usually chimerical—and the likelihood that many patients in an unselected caseload of a comprehensive community mental health center will receive greater benefit from group approaches as opposed to individual approaches.

Figure 1 indicates a ranking on a circumplex model around the two axes of control and *expectation* of the various group psychotherapy offerings of the Denver community mental health program.

Group therapies to the right of the vertical axis are characterized by increasing degrees of control. That is, the therapist or therapists place demands upon the patient's behavior during the group process. Not only is the time and place of meeting controlled by the therapist, but the therapist also adopts a generally more active, vigorous, and structuring stance than is true for the therapies to the left of the vertical axis.

Likewise, therapies above the horizontal axis are marked by increasing expectation from the therapist that the patients involved in the group experience will not only hold their own or get worse less slowly than might otherwise happen, but also will materially improve in their feelings, thoughts or behavior as a result of the group therapy experience. To discuss each of these in turn, we will first examine those in the upper right quadrant: group therapies

FIGURE 1

A Circumplex Model of Classification of Group Psychotherapies

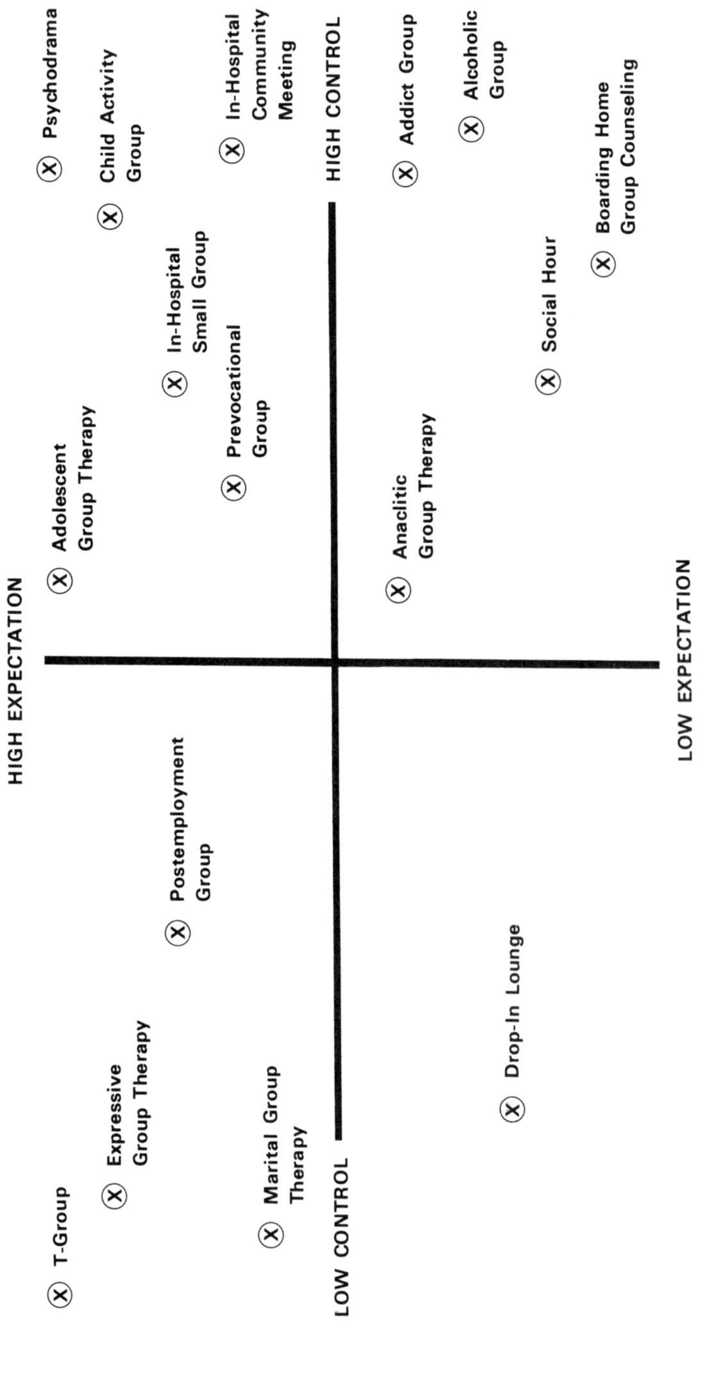

HIGH EXPECTATION

LOW EXPECTATION

HIGH CONTROL

LOW CONTROL

- (X) Psychodrama
- (X) Child Activity Group
- (X) In-Hospital Community Meeting
- (X) Addict Group
- (X) Alcoholic Group
- (X) In-Hospital Small Group
- (X) Boarding Home Group Counseling
- (X) Prevocational Group
- (X) Social Hour
- (X) Adolescent Group Therapy
- (X) Anaclitic Group Therapy
- (X) Postemployment Group
- (X) Drop-In Lounge
- (X) Expressive Group Therapy
- (X) Marital Group Therapy
- (X) T-Group

characterized by relatively high level of control and expectation.

The in-hospital community meeting is both psychotherapy and sociotherapy. Because the group is large (30 to 50 people is not unusual in many settings where hospital and day hospital patients and staff are combined), the process is quite different from small group therapy, and the expectations and behaviors of the therapist are changed. Control is exerted by therapeutic personnel within the group and is frequently necessitated by the uncontrolled affect or the difficult-to-understand verbalization or behavior of seriously ill patients in the hospital and day hospital setting. The community meeting is very stressful for many patients who suffer greatly from the feeling of exposure in talking about themselves before so many other people. Since the group is so large, however, it allows the responsibility of "carrying" the process to be widely diffused among the patients and staff, resulting in a compensatory lowering of pressure on any one individual. It allows patients to see staff, as well as other patients, and cope with difficult or disturbing behaviors of other individuals in the group. The in-hospital community meeting functions as a leveling device to promote egalitarianism and a sense of shared plight among the participating patients. Because of the size of the group and the limit on time, even with daily therapeutic community meetings, no one patient can receive a great deal of attention without severely compromising the needs of others in the group.

In contrast, the small group therapy conducted

within a hospital or day hospital setting, involving a subgroup of the patients, is characterized by a lower level of control and a higher level of expectation. In a hospital, small group therapy generally exhibits the characteristics of outpatient therapy. There is naturally much more focus on the relevance of the hospital experience, the development of insight arising from interaction with other patients and staff, and planning of posthospital adjustment.

Child activity groups involve the utilization of activity and the exploration of new experiences as a modality for helping children learn to trust a significant adult figure, to resolve conflict by discussion and compromise, and to learn adaptive skills useful in the dominant culture. This method is characterized by a high degree of control by the adult leader, who usually insists upon consensual decision-making on the part of the children prior to the initiation of any activity. He also controls their behavior in public settings, not allowing aggressive or disruptive episodes. The expectation level is also high, with the anticipation that even emotionally ill children are capable of learning by experience to behave more adaptively towards adults, to feel more comfortable with themselves, to resolve their difficulties more effectively with their peers, and to increase their domain of comfortable mastery within the community.

Psychodrama has a moderately high degree of control. Definite rules are set down, and the director shapes and molds the behavior of the psychodrama participants. It is also a method with a very high level of expectation, which assumes that people not only are capable of talking about significant life events and feelings, but also can re-experience them in the psychodrama situation, and, in the process, learn more about themselves and more effective ways of dealing with themselves and other people.

Adolescent group therapy likewise tends to have a high level of expectation, but a considerable degree of control is exerted by the adult therapist. The therapist tends to be more active and to guide and shape the therapeutic process much more than would be true for group therapy with neurotic adults.

The prevocational group is a psychiatric rehabilitation modality involving individuals who, because of their interpersonal and intrapsychic problems, have had difficulty in adapting to work situations. It prepares them for the process of seeking a job, the interview, and the task of going to work. The prevocational group is characterized by a moderate level of control and a moderate level of expectation.

Moving to the right lower quadrant, we find the group methods characterized by a relatively high level of control on the part of the staff, but relatively low expectation levels.

Anaclitic group therapy is a small group technique designed to utilize the group experience to meet the dependent and nurturance needs of seriously dependent individuals who experience difficulty adapting to their life situation because of the intensity and extent of their dependency strivings. Group therapy may be an effective modality for vitiating the strength of some of these strivings, allowing the patient to have somewhat more healthy interpersonal relationships outside of group therapy. It may also assist the patient to sustain a more adult adjustment on a day-by-day basis.

Successful group therapies for addicts and alcoholics are characterized by a high degree of control by the staff. Extremely close supervision of behavior and drug use are necessary, particularly with addicts, utilizing regular urine tests in the case of hard narcotic addiction. Most clinicians tend—probably erroneously—to have a relatively low level of expectation for alcoholics and addicts, and the group approaches often reflect this. Beginning group therapy for most alcoholics and addicts should provide, in effect, an opportunity for the exchange of alibis, with interpersonal distance, that characterizes these subcultures, taking place in a setting where alcohol or other drugs are not necessary to sustain the comfort and safety of the group situation. As treatment progresses, many alcoholics and addicts are able to move to other group therapies with a lower degree of control and a higher degree of expectation.

Social hour is our local name for a large group aftercare modality utilized in the comprehensive community mental health center of the Denver Department of Health and Hospitals. It is a weekly half-day experience for chronic psychiatric patients, characterized by high control and low expectation. Activities in the social hour consist of a blend of patient government, resocialization, remotivation, and recreation therapy. There is a use of discussion, games, business meetings, singing and dancing, and other activities to encourage interpersonal relationships and to minimize regression on the part of isolated patients.

Group counseling conducted by Visiting Nurses in boarding homes housing ex-psychiatric patients constitutes a modality with high control, but low expectation. The patients are expected to attend these sessions and are given very little degree of individual choice by the boarding home operator and the Visiting Nurse as to whether they will attend. They are characteristically patients who have shown many of the signs of the institutional or social breakdown syndrome and have been returned to the community after five to thirty years in a state hospital setting.

The upper left quadrant consists of therapies marked by low control on the part of the staff and a high expectation level. The postemployment group provides a continuity of group experience for individuals moving from the prevocational group into active employment. It focuses on the interpersonal and intrapsychic dilemmas experienced by the psychiatric patient in assuming and reentering the central life role as a wage earner. Marital group therapy is characterized by low degree of control and usually a modulated expectation on the part of the staff. Marital problem groups tend to be active and stormy, but many practitioners view the typical outcome with some reserve.

Expressive group therapy constitutes a relatively low control paradigm, in that the therapist tends not to direct the behavior or verbalization of the patients within the group and adopts a relatively passive, empathic and nonjudgmental, occasionally

interpretive stance. Expressive group therapy focuses on the process of the group, as well as generic
content expressed by individual group members. The
expectation level, in terms of the ability of the individuals to work in therapy and their ability to utilize therapy experience for change, is generally high.

T-group, sensitivity and encounter groups, are
characterized by low control and high expectation.
These groups generally direct themselves to increasing the quality of humanness in people who are essentially "normal." There have been experiments,
however, in the utilization of T-group and other
human relations training devices with psychiatric
patients with some reported successes.

A drop-in lounge is operated by some community-
based generic mental health teams in comprehensive
community mental health centers. This room is staffed
by one or more staff members—either professional or
subprofessional. Patients are encouraged to come if
they should experience some adaptational failure during the course of the week. The process in the drop-
in lounge may be a dyadic transaction, simple socialization, or at times, a kind of informal group therapy
characterized by extremely low control and relatively
low expectation.

Family therapy is the newest addition to the
group psychotherapies. To the extent that one recognizes the importance of the family as the primary group sustaining and reinstituting normative
behavior of its members, the importance of family
therapy must be recognized. There is no doubt from
the personal experience of the author and from a

review of the literature, that family therapy is an extremely powerful technique.

Unfortunately, the majority of practitioners in community mental health settings today do not have adequate training in family therapy. The community mental health center must set about to train its own staff in family therapy, and the administrator must anticipate that this requires constant effort and reinforcement. Many mental health practitioners find it extremely stressful to sit with a family; it is much more difficult to evade affective interchange, to side-step important psychological issues or to cloud them in hyperintellectualized dynamic formulations. The family is alive, interacts, affect flows. The therapist must cope with a constant array of crises, unexpected events, and sharp confrontations. Since some people who go into the mental health trades are somewhat tender, they often feel very bruised by the goings-on in family therapy. Many of them have been trained in overideational theoretical systems so they frequently are baffled by the myriad events in a single family interview and are unable to translate them into some kind of dynamic formulation that has the elegance they have been led to expect. While every community mental health practitioner need not necessarily be able to comfortably and effectively conduct family therapy, every practitioner must know when it is indicated and be capable of utilizing this resource within his own setting.

For adolescent behavior problems, for many schizophrenic illnesses, for many of the psychiatric problems

of children, and for many of the sexual perversions,
family therapy is in all likelihood the treatment of
choice for the majority of patients.

Sociotherapies

The author defines sociotherapy as peer acceptance combined with confrontation, utilized to en-
force compliance to normative expectations of the
social group. In sociotherapy the activity of fellow
patients is paramount; the mental health practitioner is of secondary importance.

Maxwell Jones (1962) has played a prominent role
in calling the attention of contemporary psychiatry
to the effect of peer group expectations. American
psychiatry's preoccupation with intrapsychic processes, and with the fascinating and complex body of
psychoanalytic theory, delayed American interest in
the effect of reference groups on the expression and
resolution of psychological conflicts.

All group therapy—both unrelated and family
therapy—contains aspects of sociotherapy. Participants express their expectations of each other and
set forth their value systems in the verbal interchange of the group process. While the therapist is
the only member of the group paid for his time, his
role in effective group therapy is often less crucial
than that of the patient community.

In all psychiatric treatment endeavors, there is
also a kind of sociotherapy going on beyond the ken
of the practitioner, as the patient interacts with
family, friends, work group, and other affiliational
groupings. But it is in the therapeutic community,

within the context of the hospital and day hospital settings, that sociotherapy reaches its most clearly identifiable form. For here, it is possible to limit to some extent the variables impinging upon the patient and to focus upon the culture of the patient-staff community as a potent factor in treatment. A basic concept of the therapeutic community holds that the most psychiatrically ill patient continues to respond to significant others in his life space, and as a result of these interactions, he may have significant emotional experiences which mitigate the severity of his symptoms. The patient may also experience destructive encounters that further impair his self-esteem and encourage him to rely upon pathological and regressive modes of coping with the environment and with himself. Several features characterize most sociotherapeutic treatment settings:

1. There is deliberate blurring of status and hierarchical distinctions between staff members of various disciplines and between patients and staff. This is usually expressed nonverbally through the abandonment of uniforms on the part of the nurses and the utilization of first names on the part of all staff members.

2. Contemporaneity is emphasized in interaction between staff and patients and between patients. Focus is upon the here and now, the interpersonal and intrapsychic events that occur within the present life space of the patient.

3. The therapeutic community meeting, involving all members of the staff and patient community, is a mainstay of the sociotherapeutic experience. An attempt is made in this large group setting to encour-

age free communication, to further weaken or dis-
solve status distinctions, and to reemphasize that all
behavior is purposive, meaningful, and the responsibility of the individual who is involved in the behavior.

4. Confrontation tends to become a predominant
interpersonal behavior on the part of the staff and
patients alike. This is in line with the general sociotherapeutic emphasis on assuming responsibility for
one's behavior, eschewing evasion of it through psychoanalytic or other psychodynamic explanation of
motivations.

5. Sociotherapeutic communities tend to be mili-
tantly antiregressive. Individuals who cannot or will
not heed these strictures against regressive behavior
often suffer punitive reprisal on the part of the
larger community.

6. The environment is more stressful for the staff
because of the abandonment of their positions of
personal and professional privilege due to the weak-
ening of status and hierarchical distinctions. The
stress on the staff is lessened, however, because of
the wide diffusion of responsibility among the staff
and patient community.

Milieu Therapy

This term milieu therapy means different things
to different people, and the concept is often so glob-
al that it is difficult to discuss. Like the concept of
sociotherapy, milieu therapy emphasizes that the
total experience of the patient is relevant in determining his improvement or lack of improvement. In
its purest sense, it includes the following concepts:

1. The environment should be protective and non-punitive.

2. Attitudes and behavior of personnel should be prescribed by the responsible clinician in order to provide corrective emotional experiences for the patient.

3. Activity should be prescribed by the responsible clinician to provide for the expression of instinctual strivings and to reinforce premorbid defensive patterns.

4. Staff attitudes, patient activities, and other features of the environment (such as degree of freedom allowed the patient, whether visitors are permitted, weekend passes, etc.) should be based upon a comprehensive psychiatric examination which attempts to develop a concept of the genetic antecedents of the present psychosocial disequilibrium. Prescribed milieu therapy is essentially based, then, upon a disease model, operating out of a kind of "antitoxin" concept: If the patient has experienced rejection from significant others in his life and has become depressed because of it, the therapeutic attitude on the part of the staff might be to show active friendliness, and the activity program might involve pleasurable activities which produce products which can be praised by staff members. In operation, the main problem with the concept of milieu therapy is that it is a highly theoretical and intellectualized model, based on reductionistic theories of human motivation and illness, and does not take into account the wide range of variability in the execution of attitude and behavior therapy on the part of psychiatric personnel.

Biological Therapies

Although biological treatment has characteristically occupied a position of low esteem within the American psychiatric establishment, it seems clear that the greatest advances in the public treatment of the major psychiatric illnesses have been due to advances in biological treatment methods.

1. Electroconvulsive therapy is rarely used in community psychiatric practice today. It would seem to be the treatment of choice only for psychotically depressed individuals who do not respond to antidepressant medication or whose discomfort or suicidal danger is so great that delay is felt to be unwarranted. Under similar circumstances of life-threatening symptomatology, the utilization of electric shock therapy in catatonic schizophrenia may be indicated, though rarely.

2. Insulin-coma therapy and insulin subcoma would seem to have no place in community psychiatric practice at the present time.

3. Metrazol, Indoklon, and CO_2 inhalation would also be out of place in community psychiatric practice at the present time.

4. Pharmacotherapy is a major part of the therapeutic armamentarium of the community psychiatric practitioner. In spite of this, most psychiatrists are inadequately prepared by their residency training for the proper prescription and supervision of psychoactive drugs.

A comprehensive review of pharmacotherapy is not within the scope of this book though certain comments will be offered. The minor tranquilizers,

while useful for short-term administration to severely anxious outpatients, have major hazards in
terms of their addictive potential. They are, by and
large, overprescribed by general practitioners, nonpsychiatric specialists, and psychiatrists alike. They
have little usefulness beyond the initial days or weeks
of treatment, and prolongation of the use of minor
tranquilizers beyond a one month period should receive very skeptical review. "Vistaril" does not seem
to share this characteristic for habituation and/or
addiction.

The major tranquilizers, consisting primarily of
the phenothiazine group, have irrefutable value for
major psychiatric morbidity. Certain of them may
also be used for the extremely anxious, neurotic
outpatient, and the resultant increase in comfort
may prove useful in reinforcing the motivation of
the patient to follow-through on the recommendation for psychiatric treatment (Whittington, Zahourek, & Grey, 1969). Again, more patients take phenothiazine medication at any point in time in any
mental health center than actually need to do so. It
has been demonstrated by a previous study
(Hornstra and Wilkinson, 1966) that about half of
the patients currently receiving phenothiazines
could be discontinued without any harmful effects.

The antidepressant medications are somewhat less
effective than many of us hoped when they were
first introduced. In moderate to severe depressions,
however, they are clearly superior to placebo; imipramine would seem to be the most effective and
least noxious substance available currently (Heller,
Zahourek, & Whittington, 1970).

Sedatives should be used with extreme caution in psychiatric patients. Purposive and nonpurposive overdoses are an ever-present danger. In addition, the characteristic of all sedatives (with the possible exception of chloral hydrate and methaqualone) to reduce rapid eye movement in sleep poses some major theoretical problems. If dreaming, as manifested by REM sleep, has an important function in conflict resolution and tension reduction in both normal and ill personalities, the pharmacologic repression of dreaming would seem to be contraindicated in psychiatric patients.

Stimulant drugs, such as amphetamine and dextro-amphetamine, should be used with caution because of the habituating and toxic properties of these drugs. Ritalin does not have the toxic side effects, nor does it seem to have as great a propensity for habituation or increased tolerance; it should be used, however, only with clear indications and only for a circumscribed time.

5. Electrostimulation (sleep therapy) does not seem to have any valid application in community psychiatric practice.

6. Twilight sleep, a much used pharmacotherapy during the second World War, is rarely used in community psychiatric practice today. It may have some usefulness in acute stress reactions but runs the risk of encouraging regression and delaying conflict resolution.

7. Narcoanalysis, utilizing intravenous amytal or other sedative drugs, is used occasionally for diagnostic purposes in community psychiatric practice.

Behavioral Therapies

Semantic confusion pervades this category. For the purposes of this discussion, we shall focus on the following examples:

1. "Behavior Therapy" is a technique involving suggestion, relaxation, and an attempt to detoxify psychonoxious stimuli by mastery through fantasy. The claims for behavior therapy have been great, and proponents of this particular approach feel that it is the first scientifically validated psychotherapy. The results reported in the literature cannot be ignored, and it seems clear that in the years ahead more community psychiatric practitioners will attempt to learn about and practice behavior therapy.

2. A variety of approaches utilizing learning theory to reinforce positive behavior ("healthy behavior") and not to reward or to punish negative behavior ("unhealthy behavior") have been experimented with in recent years. The use of a token economy in chronic schizophrenic populations in state hospitals and with psychotic, mentally retarded, and brain-damaged children have yielded striking results.

3. Psychiatric rehabilitation is currently in a phase of active growth and reformulation. Historically, the federal rehabilitation program has focused on counseling and training services for individuals with physical handicaps. Early attempts to apply rehabilitation practice to psychiatric populations, then, operated essentially out of this model. Psychiatric rehabilitation specialists have become increas-

ingly aware that a much broader and richer understanding of motivation and the learning of successful
instrumental behavior must be employed. Psychiatric
rehabilitation programs focus not only on instrumental, work-related behavior, but also upon peer
relationships, employer-employee relationships, utilization of leisure time, recreation, and so forth. Many
psychiatric patients experiencing major morbidity
have either never learned or else have forgotten
through disuse, a wide range of interpersonal, social,
and instrumental skills which are necessary for living
in contemporary American society. Current rehabilitation philosophy also operates out of the well-
documented conclusion that the removal of symptoms
and the resultant increased comfort of the patient
does not by itself necessarily increase adaptational
competency or improve instrumental functioning.
Consequently, the psychiatric rehabilitation counselor must become an active partner with the clinician
in attempting to return the patient to fully adequate
personal, social, and vocational behavior.

Situational Modification

American psychiatry has tended to look down its
nose at situational modification, seeing it as pallia-
tive or somehow peripheral to the real concern of
psychodynamically-oriented psychotherapy. Yet, the
community psychiatric practitioner is constantly
concerned with how to decrease situational stress
and increase situational support for the psychiatrically ill individual.

Decreasing situational stresses frequently challenges the ingenuity of the community psychiatric practitioner. If these stresses are interpersonal, he may find it necessary to intervene directly into the dyadic or family transaction to discourage and inhibit behavior of significant others which he believes is detrimental to the patient. He may strive to simply isolate the patient from this behavior by prescribing hospitalization, day hospital treatment, temporary separation from the family, re-employment if the individual is a nonworking housewife, or enrollment in school. The basic theory is that if one cannot do away with the psychonoxious interpersonal behaviors, then a reduction of the number of hours per week that the patient is exposed to such influences will reduce the situational stress.

Financial problems constitute a major situational stress with many individuals seen in a community psychiatric practice. An extremely effective working relationship with the welfare department is necessary if the community psychiatric practitioner is to be able to move quickly to reduce financial stress. Equally effective relationships with the Office of Economic Opportunity programs in major metropolitan areas will also allow the community psychiatric practitioner to reduce stress by helping the patient receive legal and consumer advice concerning pressures from creditors.

The poor characteristically have many legal problems. The community mental health practitioner must have available either within his own center, or in other community agencies, legal advice and assistance without charge if he is to successfully reduce situational stress for many of his patients.

The demands of dependent children are a major stress for many women. Availability of day care centers, preschool programs, summer camp and activity programs, and so forth are necessary if the community psychiatric practitioner is to be effective in reducing stresses for emotionally ill mothers.

Unemployment or underemployment are major problems for many men attempting to continue as responsible heads of families, despite psychiatric symptoms. The ability to utilize a specialized psychiatric rehabilitation program within the comprehensive community mental health center and to use existing community employment programs is essential if the needs of the psychiatrically ill male population are to be properly served.

Many patients seen in a community mental health center are also plagued by poor housing conditions, bad sanitation, an abundance of rats, attacks on their children at the local playground, and so forth. The community psychiatric practitioner must understand the social control—including health and housing control—systems within his community and have access to their services if he is to act as an effective advocate for his patient.

Situational supports frequently must be deployed by the community mental health practitioner as he develops and implements a treatment plan for his patient. Homemaker Services exist in most large American cities. The placement of a trained and supervised subprofessional in the patient's home, to assist with housekeeping and child care tasks, can be very supportive. This direct supplementation of the adequacy of the mother may be crucial: It not only offers situational support and relieves situational stress, but also provides a model of role adequacy which may result in some learning on the part of the patient.

The Visiting Nurse Service and Public Health Nurse are the most important resources in many American communities for extending situational supports. The visiting nurse is a pragmatist who, for many years, has been utilizing the principles that we have recently discovered in community mental health practice. These vigorous and effective women can be enormously useful in providing situational supports for mothers and also can provide direct assistance to children in the home. Their effectiveness is limited, however, when assisting adult males in the home situation.

A number of community mental health programs are utilizing subprofessionals, referred to as indigenous mental health workers, mental health aides, community workers, program aides, etc. These persons are very helpful in a community mental health program, since they make available to the patient someone of a similar ethnic and socioeconomic background who can serve as the patient's advocate, collaborator and assistant, confidant, and identity model. In the case of the school-age child, situational stress can often be minimized and situational support extended through the cooperation of public school personnel.

Community mental health centers have been less interested, and consequently less successful, in developing strategies for reducing situational stress and increasing situation supports for adult males, than for women and children. Professions always inherit, to some extent, the biases of the culture in which they are imbedded. In our society, men are expected to be strong, not to cry, and to keep a stiff upper lip in the face of adversity. In contrast, women are seen to be vulnerable to stress, as are children, and needy and deserving of special consideration and support. The psychiatric professions have shown a distinct preference to working with individuals who are essentially passive and utilize rumination and verbal interaction as a way of coping with problems, as opposed to the utilization of direct behavior. And, it must be admitted that, until quite recently, psychiatric professions attracted many men whose life style was passive, and whose comfort with and desire to associate with aggressive males was somewhat impaired. Again, in our culture—at least until quite recently—one would not expect the most aggressive and assertive males to be attracted to a care-giving profession, since such occupations have characteristically been viewed as being suitable for women, or for men with "feminine" characteristics.

Other Therapies

It is impressive to look at the variety of intervention strategies that mental health practitioners have come to utilize. Only two others, however, will be mentioned:

1. Hypnotherapy has a definite place in community psychiatric practice. Hypnosis may be used as an adjunct in psychotherapy which is either expres-

sive or supportive in nature. In the former instance, hypnosis is used in an attempt to breach the repressive barrier and recover unconscious material that can be used in the therapeutic process. In the latter instance, hypnosis is used to reinforce suggestion, facilitating the removal of specific symptoms. It is little used, however, probably because the nonauthoritarian bent of the typical community mental health practitioner makes it difficult for him to assume the stance of the hypnotherapist. In amnestic states, hysterical aphonias, and for a variety of patients with strong needs for magical relief of symptoms and with a strong belief in the potency of the therapist, hypnotherapy has something significant to offer.

2. Transactional analysis has been brought to our attention by the works of Berne (1964). Transactional analysis is a fresh, contemporaneous, decidedly American attempt to conceptualize, and develop a treatment strategy for, character pathology. It views the frozen or repetitious maladaptive behavior patterns of individuals in an interpersonal context, emphasizing that reciprocal behaviors are necessary to reinforce and reward maladaptive personality style. The basic point of view of transactional analysis can be carried forth in any of the psychotherapies, sociotherapies, or behavioral therapies as outlined above. Transactional analysis is a relevant and contemporary approach to the problem of understanding character pathology, which has so plagued psychiatric theorists and practitioners over the years. Its freshness, the clarity and communicability of its theoretical concepts, and the power of its "secret language," make it potentially useful for many of the

kinds of psychiatric problems that the community mental health practitioner must face.

The Setting

Any of these therapies may take place within the traditional psychiatric settings of inpatient, outpatient, and transitional therapy settings. The term "outpatient treatment" is really meaningless; one must say what kind of treatment, to what purpose, and executed by whom before one has any idea of what outpatient treatment means. The same is true for psychiatric hospitalization, for day hospital, and so forth. For example, some psychiatric hospital treatment experiences are utilized primarily to provide intensive individual psychotherapy. In contrast, some outpatient treatment programs employ a sociotherapeutic model for many of their patients.

The number of psychiatric beds believed to be necessary to serve a population of 100,000 people varies widely. New York State, for example, has many more psychiatric beds than does California, with roughly equivalent populations. In many communities, hospital treatment is greatly overutilized, and the number of beds excessive to real needs. The tendency of third-party payment plans to reimburse inpatient care more liberally than outpatient service undoubtedly contributes to this trend. Because of the high expense of hospitalization, most community mental health centers attempt to minimize bed occupancy. Concern over the subtle encouragement of regression and the covert sanctioning of the mental patient role compel the community psychiatrist to use inpatient care with considerable restraint. Figure 2 indicates alternatives to hospitalization available and encouraged in the Denver program.

In summary, the purpose of the evaluation is to decide which of these therapies may be useful in changing the patient in the direction desired by him, and/or significant others in his life, and/or by the treating persons. In addition to deciding the type of therapy, the evaluation process must decide the setting in which that therapy may most effectively be performed. In general, the complexity of the evaluation process should be a function of the number of treatment alternatives that are available within the particular context.

In deciding upon treatment, the cost-benefit issue must remain paramount in the community psychiatric practitioner's mind. The next chapter will discuss these issues from the slightly different standpoint of treatment careers.

FIGURE 2

Alternatives to Hospitalization

Reason for Hospitalization	Alternative
Reduce Situational Stress	
Interpersonal Conflict —————→	Family Therapy
	Separation
	Hotel
	Vacation
Economic ————————→	Welfare Aid
Role Demands——————→	Sick Leave
	Foster Care for Children
Increase Situational Supports	
Reassurance	Daily Phone Contact with Therapist
	Daily Brief Clinic Visit
	Visiting Nurse Service
Tangible Assistance	Homemaker
	Household Help
	Boarding Home or other Foster Living
	Situation
Peer Support	Group Therapy
	Family Therapy
Evaluation	
Behavioral Evaluation—————→	Home Visit
	VNS Evaluation
	Obtain Information from Welfare, Court,
	etc.; Interagency Conference
Physical Illness Issues——————→	Most except major CNS evaluations (i.e.,
	pneumoencephalogram) can be done as
	outpatient
Treatment	
Medication Administration and——→	Injectable (Prolixin)
Supervision	VNS Supervision
	Daily Clinic visit to receive Rx
	(as, Thorazine Spansule q.d.)
Socialization—————————→	Social Hour
	Group Rx
	Use of community socialization
	opportunities
Pleasurable Activity—————→	Social Hour
	Use of Community Resources

FIGURE 2—Continued

Alternatives to Hospitalization

Reason for Hospitalization	Alternative
Reinstitute Premorbid Behavior Patterns	Homemaker VNS Structured activity schedule Use of relatives as adjunct therapists
Legitimation of Patient Role	Verbal Formulation by Clinician to Patient and Relatives
24-hour Crisis Help	Use of Emergency Room Crisis Team and/or Primary Outpatient Clinician
Psychotherapy	Outpatient Psychotherapy
Sociotherapy (peer confrontation and enforcement of compliance to normative expectations)	Therapist activity and clear statement of expectations "Checking" on behavior by third party: VN, Welfare, Probation Officer, significant other, home visits by mental health worker and/or primary clinician Family Therapy
ECT	ECT on day-patient status
Protection of Patient from Self (suicide)	Instruction of spouse and/or other significant persons Homemaker Collect all toxic medications Have razors and guns locked up Partial hospitalization during times when at-home supervision is not possible
Protection of Others from Patient	Chemical Restraint Jail

CHAPTER IV

Treatment Careers

IN A SYSTEM which has the multiple treatment options of a comprehensive community mental health center, clinical decision-making becomes a vital function. Such a decision-making process may be facilitated by a concept of treatment careers or alternative "processing" options, helping the individual clinician clarify his responsibility in making such critical decisions.

The flow chart (Figure 1) is a beginning conceptualization of a systems approach to the clinical program of a comprehensive community mental health center. From the upper left corner, a patient presents himself to the clinician in a comprehensive community mental health center, and the beginning processes of a psychiatric evaluation are conducted to determine if psychiatric symptomatology exists. At this decision-making point (labeled A) the clinician must make a multifactorial judgment that is—as was discussed in Chapter II—not amenable to full quantification at the present time. In general, areas of functioning that are appraised in arriving at a health-sickness rating or index of psychosocial decompensation, are as follows:

1. Subjective discomfort and symptomatic behaviors

2. Adequacy of role performance and instrumental functioning

3. Intactness of ego functioning, i.e., adaptative capacities such as judgment, memory, ability to delay impulses, etc.

4. Interpersonal relationships

If the individual is judged not to have psychiatric symptoms, but has still presented himself or has been presented to a mental health practitioner in a comprehensive community mental health center, one must presume that some problem in living exists. More individuals experiencing psychological reactions to situational problems are seen in initial psychiatric evaluations because of the increasing availability and citizen awareness of comprehensive community mental health centers. If the answer to this question (at point B in the diagram) is positive, the clinician should discharge his responsibility as a caregiver by referring the individual to the appropriate resource, either within the comprehensive community mental health center or in some other agency. For example, a woman whose baby had been bitten by a rat in a tenement might appear very distraught in the emergency room of a general hospital and might find her way to, or be referred to, a psychiatric crisis team. While some degree of understanding and support could be given during the interview, the appropriate course of action would be

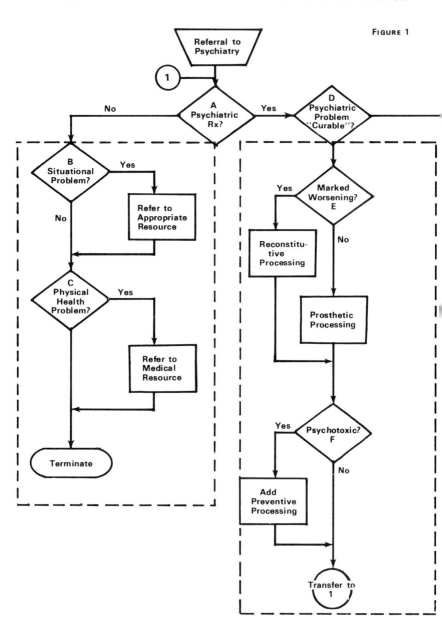

FIGURE 1

DISPOSITION-REFERRAL BRANCH   "NO-CURE" BRANCH

Flow Chart: Treatment Career

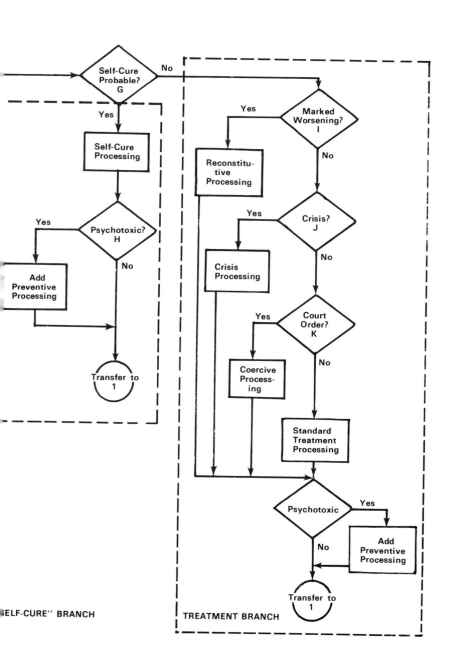

"SELF-CURE" BRANCH   TREATMENT BRANCH

to assist the woman in making contact with the City
Housing Inspection Office, in an attempt to gain
legal sanctions to force the landlord to improve her
physical surroundings. At this interface between the
community mental health practitioner and the community, the role of clinician merges imperceptibly
with that of social problem-solver and humanitarian. Most comprehensive community mental health
centers have found it advantageous to have subprofessional and nontraditional personnel available to
assist in the process of situational amelioration,
since this is a task not particularly well performed
by the traditional mental health disciplines, nor is
their training and expensive time required to deal
with such problems.

One of the ironies of modern-day life is that a fair
number of people with physical health problems
define their difficulties as psychological or have had
them defined by others as psychological and present
themselves to a community mental health practitioner. An example of this would be the older person
without a prior psychiatric history, who develops a
steadily more severe depression as the initial symp-
tom of a covert malignancy; also, the individual
whose anxiety symptoms and restlessness are associated with increased function of the thyroid gland.
Where the presenting complaints of the individual
are not felt to be primarily psychiatric symptoms,
but judged to represent a physical health problem
(point C in the diagram), referral to the appropriate
medical resource should be initiated.

There is no real consensus at present about the
importance of a comprehensive physical examina-

tion as part of a psychiatric evaluation. Our "public morality" tells us that this is good idea; in practice, however, most private psychiatrists and many public community mental health centers indicate that we do *not* place great value on a routine physical appraisal. It is certainly true that only an infinitesimal number of cases of organic illness are discovered by routine physical appraisal. A more rational approach would probably be to have the initial decision-making (performed at points A, B, and C) conducted in all cases by a well-trained and experienced psychiatrist. This would be practicing our philosophical point of view that psychiatrists are useful in the diagnosis and treatment of psychological problems because they bring a balanced view of not only psychological and social, but also organic factors to bear upon an understanding of the patient's difficulties. Most psychiatrists do not act as if they believed this was true, and most agencies do not deploy their resources in a way which indicates they are convinced. This is an important area for program evaluation and research: to determine if there *are* advantages to the patient in having a psychiatrist conduct the initial appraisal.

Multiphasic screening programs, such as those in use at the Kaiser-Permanente Medical Group in California, offer considerable promise for a low cost, more sensitive screening device for physical illness. Where such facilities are available, they may well substitute for the routine physical examination conducted in some psychiatric settings. The importance that one places in program planning on the physical examination, and the amount of resources that can be justifiably deployed in accomplishing the goals of an adequate physical appraisal, would be determined by the characteristics of the population served. A comprehensive community mental health center serving the central city of a major metropolitan area, for example, would in its emergency and hospital service have a very high percentage of individuals experiencing disorders of thinking, feeling, or behaving that are related to organic illness states. In contrast, a clinic serving a middle-class white suburb would find significant physical illness in a very small percentage of their clientele.

If the answer of the decision-making process A is yes, the clinician must next ask himself whether from our available store of knowledge about psychiatric states and our available change technology, the problem would seem to be "curable" (point D). The humanitarian impulses and omnipotent fantasies of the clinician come most powerfully into play here. In many settings, the decision is *rarely* made that the probability of cure is low or absent.

In the patient has been ill for more than two years, with significant impairment in two or more of the areas listed as part of the decision-making schedule at point A, and has had prior treatment by a competent practitioner and/or agency, presumptive assignment should be made to the "untreatable" category. As manpower resources expand in a specific community mental health program, the criteria for designation as untreatable becomes less rigid. With fixed resources and expanding demands for service, however, a significant proportion of individuals seeking treatment in a new community mental health center should probably be assigned to the untreatable category if the needs of the community and individuals more amenable to treatment are to be met.

If the individual is experiencing a rapid worsening in his general level of psychosocial adequacy (point E), the decision may be to institute reconstitutive processing, in spite of the poor prognosis for successful outcome of treatment. Reconstitutive processing —such as that offered to a chronically psychotic individual discharged from the state hospital after five years of hospital treatment, who begins to become delusional and unkempt—consists of the following:

1. Situational supports are maximized; therapy is controlling and is not permissive or nondirective.

2. Psychoactive drugs are used extensively.

3. Protection from situational stresses, by brief hospitalization if necessary, is emphasized.

4. The goal is reinstitution of preworsening level of homeostasis. The patient is told, "Once we get you functioning better, we'll decide what kind of further treatment you need."

5. Active processing is terminated as soon as the best level of recent functioning is approximated, and infrequent monitoring contacts utilizing such personnel as Visiting Nurses or mental health workers, is instituted.

If the "uncurable" patient is not experiencing a marked worsening, the mental health practitioner will usually decide upon "prosthetic processing." This involves the following elements:

1. The clinician will communicate a recognition of the severity and chronicity of the patient's illness.

Usually he will not use labels such as "schizophrenia," but will talk in nontechnical terms about the difficulty that the individual has had in living his life to his own satisfaction.

2. The clinician will pinpoint areas of disability so far as possible, such as memory deficiencies, problems in abstract thinking, slowness, delusions, and socialization impairment, and will discuss these specifically with the patient as the focus of prosthetic intervention.

3. The clinician will utilize psychoactive medication to minimize disability as much as possible.

4. The community mental health practitioner will marshal community resources to compensate for disabilities. Examples might include: (a) The appointment of a guardian in cases of impaired judgment, (b) The utilization of a social hour or other resocialization activity for socially isolated individuals, (c) The deployment of a Visiting Nurse for individuals who have impaired help-seeking behavior, in order to determine that they are ensuring, at least marginally, adequate competency in their self-care, (d) The assignment of a patient to a boarding home if self-care is judged to be inadequate, and (e) The utilization of a terminal sheltered workshop in cases of vocational impairment, but where significant residual adequacy remains to justify the utilization of the service.

In any of the "noncurable" cases, the community mental health practitioner must examine the effect of the individual's psychosocial difficulties on significant others in his life space. If the patient is actually doing psychological harm to other persons in the environment, especially if the "victims" are high risk or vulnerable individuals (children, aged, physically or mentally handicapped), intensive intervention is indicated. Mothers, marital partners, industrial supervisors, and caregiving professionsals all have great potential to become psychonoxic agents.

If the answer at point F is yes, then preventive processing will be added to reconstitutive and/or prosthetic processing. This will involve the following:

1. Family therapy, to increase the adaptive capacities of the family unit, should be the initial intervention modality in the vast majority of cases.

2. Supplementation of family resources in order to "immunize" children should be considered early: Headstart, summer camp, Homemakers, etc.

3. Direct assistance to the family in coping with the destructive members should be freely extended through the use of intermittent hospitalization, day care, Visiting Nurse Service, and so forth.

4. Marshalling all agency and community resources for intensive and sustained intervention.

5. Maximizing the controlling aspects of the therapist's behavior in order to protect the victims.

6. Medication should be used fully to control noxious symptoms.

If these approaches are unsuccessful, temporary removal of vulnerable members—placement of children in a foster home—should be considered early.

At any point where the particular processing does not seem to be adequate or appropriate, the patient should be reintroduced to the decision-making process: A new appraisal is made of symptomatology and of the appropriate and available change technology which can be brought to bear upon the individual's difficulties. In a comprehensive community mental health center, periodic reevaluation of the entire treatment load, as well as reevaluation on an ad hoc basis, should be initiated when difficulties arise or the individual's response does not seem to be appropriate.

If the answer at decision-making point D is yes, that psychiatric cure seems probable, the clinician in an overtaxed mental health center must ask himself whether *self*-cure is possible. The number of areas of impairment as well as the severity of impairment in a single area should be considered in arriving at a judgment of whether the patient is likely to recover spontaneously. For example, subjective discomfort without impairment in role adequacy, adaptive capacity, or interpersonal difficulty would be likely to heal spontaneously. Difficulties of recent onset with definable, but not catastrophic precipitants, would also be considered likely to self heal. The clinician should also ask, "Is the intrapsychic or interpersonal feedback from the presenting complaint likely to impede restitution of normality?"

If the answer at point G is yes, the client should be assigned to self-cure processing, which consists of the following features:

1. The clinician should communicate a sense of optimism to the patient.

2. A three- to six-month follow-up visit to insure adequate resolution should be structured.

3. The client should be instructed about contingencies which may arise, such as what to do in the

case of worsening, how to deal with situational stresses or crises, and so forth.

4. The clinician may prescribe minor tranquilizers on an as-needed basis if he feels they are indicated, as long as this is presented to the patient as an aid in coping with his symptoms, not as a cure or magical solution to his problems.

5. If the individual is psychotoxic, preventive processing should be added to self-cure processing.

6. In the event that the individual does not respond within the arbitrarily defined follow-up period, the patient should be reappraised at point A, and the decision-making path followed through again.

It is part of the folklore of psychiatry that many of the patients left on waiting lists recover spontaneously. Some studies even present soft data that this does actually occur. Unfortunately, many practitioners conclude, consequently, that we should keep everybody on a waiting list. What we should do instead, in the view of the author, is to maximize our capability for rational problem-solving so that we can decide *which* individuals will do better left to their own devices and which ones will only become *more* disabled and uncomfortable if subjected to a wait. It is not appropriate for a scientist or a humanitarian to allow the forces of random chance and fate to be substituted for our assumption of responsibility as rational men and clinical decision-makers.

As the diagram indicates at point H, if the individual is psychotoxic, even if self-cure is probable, preventive processing should be added. If the answer at point G is no, that self-cure is not probable, a number of possibilities should be considered.

If marked worsening is possible, reconstitutive processing should be added. If marked worsening (point I) is not likely, one should ask whether situational variables are the most prominent aspect of the current disequilibrium. If the individual's psychiatric symptomatology is a part of his response to a crisis situation—which results from an interplay of external and internal variables—the clinician should proceed on the assumption that a prompt restitution of premorbid functioning can be expected by supporting ego functioning, decreasing situational stresses, and increasing situational supports. Consequently, crisis processing is initiated: (1) the formulation is communicated to the patient that his situation is seen as a crisis and short-term intervention is planned; (2) appropriate crisis or sector psychotherapy, with situational modification as appropriate, is instituted.

The patient may have been referred to the mental health center by court order, or by some other coercive action of the social control system. In that instance, coercive processing (K) would be the treatment career of choice. Coercive treatment processing encompasses the following elements:

1. Control elements of the treatment process are maximized by actual or threatened legal sanctions.

2. The therapist has a dual responsibility—to society and to the patient—and the contract with the patient must recognize this clearly and honestly.

3. The control of socially objectionable behavior becomes the primary goal of initial treatment.

4. The incompetence of the individual to "refrain from the wrong" is implicitly accepted, and the ther-

apist becomes an auxiliary ego while the court is an auxiliary superego.

5. The teaching of ego skills—self-observation, delay of impulses, seeking of substitute impulse gratification, interpersonal competence—and enhancing social adequacy—job training, employment counseling, etc.—become major intervention foci.

In most mental health centers, fewer than half of the cases will be candidates for standard treatment processing or the traditional treatment approach of psychiatry in the United States. This reality causes the most discomfort and the most resistance to the community mental health center approach among conventionally trained mental health practitioners in the United States. Unfortunately, most of the major disciplines still train people almost exclusively in the standard American treatment processing, which emphasizes the following points:

1. The major variables are considered to be intrapsychic rather than situational.

2. Supportive aspects of the transaction are maximized and controlling aspects are minimized.

3. The therapist is seen as a helping rather than a directive agent.

In standard treatment processing, an individualized treatment plan is evolved to apply current technology, primarily dyadic psychotherapy, within the limits of available manpower, to the life problem as defined by the patient. A treatment contract with mutual responsibility and expectations on the part of patient and therapist alike is developed; deviation from the expectation of the contract is considered probable cause for terminating the therapy transaction. As in the other major treatment career blocks, preventive processing may also be necessary if the individual is felt to be psychotoxic.

This conceptualization of the responsibility of the clinician, within the system in which he works, is foreign to most mental health practitioners and strikes many as mechanistic and impersonal. The intent is quite the contrary: It is to allow the individual clinician to maximize his technical competence and his human sensibilities in the service of an individual client, within the context of the real world, with all of its limitations of availability and adequacy of technology to change human behavior, thoughts, and feelings.

In the years ahead, our feeble beginnings at understanding diagnostic and treatment systems, in an attempt to comprehend the impact of system variables upon our patients, must become more complex and more sophisticated. Until that occurs, we will not be able to achieve the kind of reproducibility, sound program evaluation, and research so needed in the community mental health field.

CHAPTER V

Treatment Continuity

CONTINUITY OF CARE has become part of the rhetoric of community psychiatry; agreement about its meaning and implementing the reality of the concept have lagged considerably behind. Our current preoccupation with treatment continuity has two roots:

A. The preexisting service delivery system has been marked by fragmentation of responsibility and authority, overspecialization of mission, and public irresponsibility. As a consequence, psychiatrically ill persons have moved from agency to practitioner to agency in the great American game called "pass the patient"; players in this game earn a point every time a most seriously ill patient is foisted on an agency with an already overburdened staff of the lowest technical competence. In the comprehensive community mental health center concept, continuity of care is proposed as an antidote to this system pathology.

B. Heavy emphasis in American psychiatric theory and practice on dyadic psychotherapy, with its accompanying myth system concerning the primacy of the interpersonal transaction and the practitioner's fantasies about his own omnipotence and central life importance to the patient, have contributed to our belief that beginning and completing therapy with the same individual practitioner is of transcending value to the patient.

In its simplest terms, continuity of care implies that the same mental health practitioner sees the patient initially, conducts the evaluation, and carries treatment through to completion. This concept appeals to the pastoral romanticism within every American, since it promises return to a simpler life where a man is a jack-of-all-trades. Certain "progressive" mental health endeavors have attempted to put this concept into practice. It does not allow for the chronicity of many psychiatric patients or the increasing repertoire of intervention strategy available (which few individual mental health practitioners are capable of mastering completely), nor does it accommodate itself to the high turnover rate in personnel which characterizes most public mental health agencies.

At a higher level of complexity, continuity of care is thought to mean the assumption and maintenance of responsibility for comprehensive care by an identifiable operating unit within a mental health agency. This envisions the assumption and maintenance of responsibility by that same *group* of professional people—the generic mental health team serving a defined population living in a geographically circumscribed area—for each patient throughout his treatment career. This sort of team, when it is backed up by specialized service elements, may go a long way towards meeting demands for comprehensiveness in care, since it is not expected that each and every team member will be fully competent in all types of psychiatric intervention. The team concept may also accommodate itself to the realities of staff turnover, since a multidisciplinary group holds final responsibility, rather than a single individual operating in isolation. The high geographic mobility of urban dwellers in America, however—approximately one-fifth of the families in American cities change their residence each year—vitiates the usefulness of this concept in the case of chronic psychiatric illness and disabilities. An even higher rate of nomadism among psychiatric patients further increases the problem, as ill individuals move with distressing regularity from the district of one mental health team to another.

One may equally conceive of continuity of care as the assumption and maintenance of responsibility for comprehensive treatment by an identifiable agency. This model offers the greatest possibility for comprehensive care, accommodates itself to geographic moves between districts within a city, and allows for the reality of staff turnover and transfer. Problems of scale, however, occur in large agencies; little technology or prior experience is available to assist in developing an adequate system for monitoring continuity of care.

In regulations governing the administration of staffing grant assistance, under the Community Mental Health Centers Program, the National Institute of Mental Health has stated that the goal of comprehensiveness of care is served when free movement of staff, patients, and records is guaranteed between all service elements—whether under single administrative direction or not—serving a defined population group. While it is clear that such movement is a necessary condition for continuity of care, adequate evidence exists to prove it is not always a guarantee for it.

To achieve continuity in the real world, the comprehensive mental health center practitioner must look to the following issues: record-keeping, monitoring of longitudinal treatment career, and linkage systems between service elements. Record-keeping is an essential but much neglected part of community mental health practice. In recent decades, service delivery systems in the public sector have tended to be preoccupied with elaborate record-keeping systems, but these have not adequately served the needs of either patients or staff. Many individuals who have chosen to risk a community mental health career have overreacted to the deficiencies in this process and/or the descriptive data-oriented record-keeping systems; they bring with them an aversion to recording data about patients or therapeutic activities.

An adequate record system is vital, however, when one recognizes the chronicity of many psychiatric illnesses. The wish of the individual practitioner to be the first and last individual to see a patient is seldom realized. The typical psychiatric patient consults multiple practitioners and agencies over a life-span. He also characteristically drops out of and reenters a single service delivery system as his condition betters and worsens. Record-keeping meets the

needs of the patient, then, by making the information and treatment experience of prior encounters
with the mental health establishment available to
the clinician at the time of reevaluation and treatment planning. In community psychiatry we cannot
afford the luxury of distrusting the work of all of
our psychiatric colleagues and insist upon completing a total evaluation every time a patient presents
himself. In the interests of economy and public accountability, we must utilize all information available from prior psychiatric encounters. We can only
do this if adequate records are available.

In the comprehensive community mental health
program of the Denver Department of Health and
Hospitals, the Psychiatric Services Admission form
is completed at the time of initial evaluation. One
copy is placed in the central hospital file, and a copy
is kept in the team file for decentralized teams. Periodic progress notes are kept on a gummed form, one
copy is placed on a preruled page in the patient's
hospital chart and another is kept in the decentralized team's chart. Whenever there is any change
in the patient's condition, any change in medication, or any change in treatment planning or strategy,
a progress note is recorded.

For patients on hospital status, a narrative
work-up covering current complaints of the patient,
past history, psychiatric examination, physical and
laboratory examination, and diagnosis and treatment
planning is dictated and placed in the chart. Such a
comprehensive evaluation is encouraged for all outpatients and day hospital patients, but is not a

mandatory requirement of record-keeping so long as the Psychiatric Services Admission form and periodic progress notes are completed.

At the time the patient is discharged from the hospital service, or terminated from outpatient or other treatment, a Treatment Termination Summary is filled out. This form was designed to provide information maximally utilizable by the subsequent clinician in understanding the treatment preceding his evaluation and in developing subsequent treatment plans.

In addition, a variety of specialized forms exist for such purposes as referral of patients for psychological testing, vocational rehabilitation services, electroenchalographic study, specialty medical consultation, etc. These are made a part of the hospital chart of the patient.

MONITORING OF THE TREATMENT CAREER

As one shifts from a dyadic, acute disease model to a chronic disease, system-oriented point of view, attention must be focused on how continuity of care is monitored. In a larger system—which will characterize most urban mental health centers in the years to come—definite institutional arrangements must be made for monitoring through administrative procedures. This will attempt to insure that attrition in transfer of patients between service elements is not excessive and also to ascertain whether personnel adequacy is sufficient to enhance continuity of care for certain categories of patients.

Whenever a patient is transferred from one service

element to another, the transferring element initiates the Continuity of Care Form. The original copy is forwarded to a central location, staffed by an individual who is designated as the Continuity of Care Coordinator. Two copies are forwarded to the recipient element, and a copy is retained in the sending element's files.

Arbitrary time limits are set for each of the categories of follow-through priority. For example, an individual seen in the Psychiatric Emergency Service following a suicide attempt of high lethality, but who is not felt to require hospitalization or can not be hospitalized because of unavailability of a bed, would probably be placed in an urgent category. If within 48 hours the Continuity of Care Coordinator has not received word from the recipient element that the patient had been seen, she will contact the recipient element by telephone and inquire about the outcome of the referral. If the patient has not been heard from, the decision whether the recipient element or the Continuity of Care Coordinator will institute outreach procedures is quickly reached.

The initial outreach procedure entails an attempt to telephone the patient and/or a responsible other. If the patient can not be reached by telephone, or if the telephone contact is unsuccessful, the Visiting Nurse Service will be asked to make a home visit to evaluate the patient's condition and attempt to reinforce motivation for continuing in psychiatric treatment. If this, too, is unsuccessful, one of the team members, nonprofessional and/or professional, will consider the desirability of making a home visit, either alone or in the company of the Visiting Nurse.

Urgent categories are usually reserved for patients who are believed potentially suicidal or harmful to others or who are experiencing an extremely rapid worsening of their psychiatric condition. A follow-through priority of "highly desirable" is utilized for individuals experiencing a psychotic illness, usually diagnosed as schizophrenic, whose condition seems to be worsening and whose illness is characterized by a significant loss of effective help-seeking behavior. Moderate follow-through priorities are utilized for more chronic psychotics or those with organic brain impairment who are not experiencing an acute worsening, but who have some impairment of help-seeking behavior. Individuals with a wide variety of neurotic and personality disorders whose behavior has characteristically been self-defeating also receive this designation.

For most patients, no mandatory follow-through is requested. Whenever the decision is made by the referring clinician to assume some responsibility for monitoring continuity of care between the service elements, the assumption is that this invasion of the right of privacy of the individual is warranted by the severity of impairment of judgment and adaptational capacity. This system does not imply an unwarranted or haphazard invasion of the privacy of individuals experiencing psychiatric illnesses.

LINKAGE SYSTEM

In addition to paper, people must move between

service elements in a comprehensive community mental health program. We have found two concepts helpful in assuring continuity of service. Most important is the principle of mandatory acceptance by the recipient element. This implies that any patient referred by an element within a comprehensive community mental health program must and will be accepted for service by the unit receiving the referral. If an outpatient team, for example, refers a patient for hospital treatment, this referral will be accepted without challenge by the inpatient staff. The same expression of confidence in the judgment of their professional peers will be shown by the outpatient team, which is required to accept a patient referred for outpatient treatment. As in all systems, errors in judgment are made and inappropriate referrals occur. Abandonment of the "reevaluation" procedure, however, which is so popular among psychiatric practitioners, results in a much higher level of responsible behavior on the part of all clinicians, avoids needless duplication of evaluation procedures, and produces a climate of trust and mutuality which is pleasant for staff and beneficial for patients.

Exchange of personnel between service elements is also an extremely important part of the linkage system. In addition to the communication opportunities that such an exchange of staff provides, it also serves as a powerful antidote to the development of "first-class" and "second-class" service elements. In our system, each outpatient team psychiatrist makes daily rounds on the inpatient and day hospital service with patients from his district. He works collaboratively with the hospital nursing and ancillary therapy staff, as well as with the psychiatric administrator of the hospital service, to develop and implement treatment plans. These efforts have eroded the old animosity and isolation which existed between outpatient and inpatient services, helped the morale of the inpatient staff, and diluted the sense of isolation of the outpatient psychiatrist. Results have also included a decrease in the readmission rate to the hospital service, an increase in effective utilization of aftercare, and a decrease in the rate of transfer to the state hospital serving Denver. In addition, each outpatient team supplies a group therapist on a twice-a-week basis. He conducts reality-oriented, posthospital planning therapy groups on the inpatient service and the day hospital service with patients from its geographic district. These beginning measures were undertaken in one comprehensive community mental health center to enhance the likelihood of continuous care. The effectiveness of these methods in achieving their goal is still moot, and undoubtedly other effective approaches will be developed in our center and elsewhere.

For all this, there is no clear demonstration that achieving continuous care results in a predictably better outcome for the typical psychiatric patient. We may find, after all of our efforts, that the energy invested in maintaining such a continuity of care system—which assumes a certain degree of incompetence on the part of the patient, that he is not able to prescribe the right service for himself at the right time—is, after all, not worth the price that we must pay. Formal evaluation efforts in our center, and undoubtedly in other comprehensive community mental health centers, should begin in the near future to provide information concerning the usefulness of continuity of care efforts.

INSTRUCTIONS, CONTINUITY OF CARE SYSTEM

I. *Purpose of System.* This system is intended to provide information to help ease the movement of patients between units and services as needed. It monitors the initiation of a transfer, the contacts made or attempted by the receiving element, and the outcome of the transfer. The information is used in making clinical decisions concerning the need to "reach out" to a patient in the community and to evaluate the adequacy of the program providing continuous care.

II. *Characteristics of the System.* The system consists of element members who transfer a patient, the Continuity of Care Coordinator (CCC), and the receiving element members responsible for continued care—usually the team leader, the team secretary, and a team clinician. A continuity of care form (Psych 82A) is used to record information needed to cover the transfer process and initiate outreach attempts.

III. *Responsibility for System Functioning.* The responsibility for providing continuous care to patients resides with the Director of Psychiatric Services. Seeing that specific patients receive the care needed is the responsibility of the *receiving element,* which presumably is the appropriate element for providing the care needed at that point in the patient's career. The transferring element has the responsibility of providing information to the receiving element and to the CCC. Responsibility for the overall system operation is delegated by the Division Director to the Director of Operations.

IV. *Transfers Covered by the System.* All transfers or referrals from one service element of the Division to another, *except* those which involve the same generic team or the same physical facility, are to be handled through the system.

Examples of transfers covered:
- —Emergency Service to Team A Inpatient or Day Care
- —Emergency Service to Team A Outpatient
- —Team A Outpatient to Team B Outpatient
- —Alcoholism Intake Unit to Team A Outpatient

Examples of transfers *not* covered:
- —Team A Inpatient to Team A Outpatient
- —Team A Inpatient to Team B Inpatient

Under specific arrangements, the system will cover *any* type of transfer occurring between the Division of Psychiatric Services and other psychiatric, social, or other agencies.

V. *Initiation of Transfer by the Sending Element.* After it has been determined that further care for a patient is to be provided by another Division element, the sending element should:

A. Notify the patient that he is to be seen by another Division element and *try to obtain his agreement to contact the new element.* In the event of a transfer outside the Division, obtain the *patient's permission* to send clinical information about him and note this on the form.

B. Complete the Continuity of Care Form (C/C), Psych 82A.

1. Enter the name of the sending element, the receiving element, the date of transfer, and the primary reason for transfer in the top section.

2. Enter the patient data as required in the second section.

3. Enter the clinical information required in the third section. *Be concise* in your description.

4. Choose an appropriate *follow-through priority,* with approximate lengths of time between origination of transfer and required follow-up as indicated below:

URGENT—Follow-up within two days, if possible.

HIGHLY DESIRABLE— Follow-up within five working days.

MODERATE—Follow-up within 10 working days.

ELECTIVE— Follow-up within 15 working days *if* judged desirable by receiving element.

OTHER— Follow-up within indicated time interval (indicate on form).

NOT REQUIRED— Form sent for information purposes only; follow-up not required.

C. Send the original (white) copy of the C/C Form to the Continuity of Care Coordinator, currently located at MHC No. 5, Denver General Hospital.

D. Send the second and third copies to the receiving element to which the patient is being referred or transferred.

E. Retain the fourth (blue) copy for the sending element's files OR the sending element's patient chart.

VI. *"Outreach" Procedures for Receiving Elements.* Within the broad outlines indicated below, each team will handle its continuity of care transfers as it deems most desirable and effective. Team leaders will prepare a written plan for handling these transfers, to be filed with the Continuity of Care section (Operations Section) and posted so it is available at the team facility. The plan will provide for screening of mail for incoming C/C forms, relay of forms to team member or secretary for checking against recent patient-contact records, initial contact of patients by telephone, writing to patients, requesting a Visiting Nurse home visit, and scheduling a home visit by a team clinician as needed. The plan will also include the carrying out of these functions if any key person in the procedure is ill, on vacation, or otherwise not available to handle incoming transfers. The following should be included in each element's written plan:

A. When an *"Urgent"* Priority Form is received:

1. If the patient has not yet been contacted, try to *telephone* the patient.

2. If there is no contact, notify the team leader.

3. Schedule a VNS or team clinician home visit immediately (telephone the VNS and follow up with a written request, signed by an M.D. on the same day).

B. When a *"Highly Desirable"* or *"Moderate"* Priority Form is received:

1. If the patient is not seen within the suspense period, try to *telephone* him.

2. If no contact is made, write the patient and again request him to contact the receiving element.

3. If there still is no contact, notify the team leader who will determine further outreach procedures, if any.

C. When an *"Elective"* Priority Form is received:

1. If the patient is not seen within the suspense period, try to *telephone* him,

2. If there is no contact, notify the team leader who will decide on further action to be taken, if any.

D. The *telephone contact* must be attempted first, in the interests of speed of contact and economy of effort. Home visits are expensive and limit the number of persons who can be contacted in any one day.

E. Suspense times are to be calculated from the *date on the form,* regardless of delays that may slow down the receipt of the form. Thus, as "Urgent" form dated May 2 and received on May 4 requires immediate action, *not* a delay until May 6.

VII. *Recording of Transfer and Outreach Information by Receiving Element.* When the final outcome has been determined, the details of the patient contact and outreach efforts are to be written *on the C/C Form;* the lower left-hand corner may be usable until the form is revised appropriately.

EXAMPLE: "Patient called in 5-24-69 for appt. on 5-27-69. No show. Telephoned patient on 5-28-69, no answer. VNS visit requested 5-28-69. Patient refused to come in. Team leader discontinued outreach 5-31-69."

Either the yellow or pink copy of the C/C Form *must be returned to the CCC at Denver General Hospital;* the other copy may be filed at the team and/or placed in the patient's chart.

VIII. *Functions of the Continuity of Care Coordinator.* The CCC will monitor the transfer information concerning each patient being moved to a new service under this system. Within two days following the expiration of the suspense period for each transfer, the CCC will check for the receipt of the pink copy of the C/C Form; if not yet received, the CCC will telephone the receiving element and inquire into the circumstances and outreach efforts undertaken.

In the event of any failure in communication concerning the transfer of a patient, such as delay of papers, loss of papers in the mail, insufficient information to effect the transfer, etc., the *CCC shall have the responsibility and authority to override established procedures and request prompt action by the receiving or sending element as needed.*

IX. *Publication of Transfer Success Rates and Associated Data.* Records of the outreach efforts made and outcomes of all transfers will be maintained in the CCC office. At intervals, transfer success rates for each element and each type of transfer will be calculated and distributed to element leaders and clinical administrators of the Division.

CHAPTER VI

Caseload Regulation
and Treatment Termination

THERE IS no more difficult task for the American mental health practitioner than to limit a patient's access to treatment. As practicing moralists and sometimes religionists, our zeal for "saving" people knows no bounds. In professional training programs, our strivings for omniscience, omnipotence, and omnisentience are stimulated, reinforced, and rewarded by the programs' faculties. These strivings are particularly appealing to the American character, with our national tendency to believe that all things are possible and just trying hard enough will make anything come true.

The reality of community mental health practice is at marked odds with these emotional preferences. In the real world, there is never enough clinical time to go around. There are always more patients who are suitable candidates for long-term individual psychotherapy than there are available long-term psychotherapy hours. No patient ever reaches a point where "just one more hour" would not have something beneficial to offer him, or at least we seem to feel this is the case.

The public mental health practitioner is free of certain constraints that affect the private practitioner's behavior. He gains no personal economic reward from the patient's remaining sick and in treatment, as does the private practitioner. It is generally easier, however, even in public practice, to continue to see a patient that one has known over a period of time than to start with a stranger with unfamiliar problems.

If the community mental health practitioner is to provide a public service to the community, and if the mental health team is to fulfill its responsibilities within the agency, constant attention must be paid to the termination of treatment. A close watch must be kept on cost-benefit issues, as well as the pressure for service from those who have not yet received *any* treatment.

The beginning of adequate caseload regulation lies in the initial interview and in the evaluation process. So long as goals are realistically formulated, clearly stated, and incorporated in the psychological contract between patient and treator, the termination of treatment can be easily arrived at by mutual consent. To the extent that goals are more ambitious than our available technology warrants, or to the extent that the goals are not formulated or are not consensually held by the patient and treator, the determination of a reasonable end point for the treatment career will be somewhat more vexing.

Generally speaking, the community psychiatric practitioner responds supportively to the patient's early communications concerning ambivalence about continuing treatment, tending to accept a decision to abandon the treatment career. This is at marked variance with the characteristic behavior of psychoanalytically-oriented private psychiatric practitioners, who tend to view such strivings as "resistance," or "flight into health." The community mental health practitioner, operating in a system that guarantees some degree of continuity and availability, can afford to be more flexible about termination. Health is health, whether it is flown into and whether it lasts one week, one year, or forever. The community psychiatric practitioner can and does tell the patient, "I'm glad you are feeling better. I think you've learned that the kind of treatment we have offered can be useful to you; and you've also learned more about ways in which you can cope with some of the life problems that caused you to become ill. If you begin to have trouble again in the future, you know where I am and how to contact me, and I hope you will feel free to do so before things get too rough for you."

In reality, then, in a community psychiatric practice the patient has actually never "terminated." "Termination" is an unfortunate fossil, growing out of the acute disease model and the concept of definitive psychotherapy. No one ever thinks of "terminating" a patient in traditional medical practice. The patient receives treatment for the complaints he brings and treatment ends, but the record and the process is in no way closed out. It is assumed by the general practitioner that the patient, after treatment for a sore throat, will not be coming back as long as his throat does not hurt, but that he may return for a throat infection or some other infection.

Similarly, the orthopedist assumes that after the fracture is healed the cast will be removed and he will not see the patient unless a subsequent accident should cause another fracture. He does not "terminate" the case, but simply places it in his inactive file. This is a very pragmatic and useful point of view for the community psychiatric practitioner, one that unfortunately is not shared by state and national agencies requesting reports of terminated outpatients.

In planning the investment of his time in a treatment course, the practitioner should remember that we have some evidence that comfort can be increased by very brief contacts between therapist and patient, and fifty-minute hours are certainly not always necessary if the goal is to help the patient be more comfortable. We also have some evidence that most rapid gains in psychotherapy occur within the first ten hours of treatment and that subsequent to that time, the learning or behavioral change curve flattens.

One of the responsibilities of the team leader is to periodically review the caseload of each team member in order to guard against unnecessary prolongation of treatment careers (this is discussed more fully in Chapter VII). Particularly for inexperienced clinicians, the temptation always exists to prolong treatment in the hopes that the "key" which has eluded the practitioner previously can be uncovered. Many community mental health practitioners are unable to distinguish between character pathology, which cannot be affected by a short or even moderate course of individual or group psychotherapy, and reactive pathology or symptoms resulting from adaptational failure. The vast majority of mental health practitioners still enter community mental health centers viewing individual psychotherapy as the treatment of choice. They evidence extremely limited capability to prescribe alternative intervention based on learning or behavior theory, which is often performed by nontraditional practitioners such as psychiatric rehabilitation counselors.

The basic stance of the practitioner should be, in most cases, that failure of a particular treatment approach over a period of some weeks indicates the abandonment of treatment or the substitution of some other approach, rather than blind persistence in and perseveration of the initially chosen methodology.

Every time a community mental health practitioner meets with the patient, he must ask himself:

Do I have evidence that this patient is continuing to improve?

If I'm not sure this patient is improving, should I end treatment, or try an alternative approach?

If I persist in this or some other alternative treatment, what do the prognostic indicators show the likelihood of a productive outcome?

If I persist in an active treatment program with this patient, how many people am I denying access to any treatment at all?

Is it really a mean thing to tell a patient that I think he is healthier now and no longer needs treatment?

Whose needs am I meeting by seeing this patient again, his or mine?

To what extent are my perfectionistic strivings leading me to continue to commit scarce resources to the treatment of this particular individual?

Am I motivated by voyeurism? Am I gaining any vicarious gratification from the relationship with this patient?

Would anything terrible happen if I told this patient I thought we needn't meet regularly for awhile, and that I might see him in a month or two to check on how he is getting along? Or might I tell him to simply call me and set up another appointment if things should begin to go badly again?

Is he really getting his money's worth for the fee that he is paying (even though it is a reduced fee, it has equal value in relationship to his available income) or is the service that he is receiving not worth the price he is paying?

By asking and attempting to answer such hard questions as these over and over again, the community psychiatric practitioner develops, with help from consultants and more senior clinicians, a balanced sense of values; he does not abandon the humanistic and individualized concerns of the traditional psychiatric practitioner, but supplements them by pragmatic issues of supply and demand, availability of resources and responsibility to a population-at-risk, in addition to a sense of accountability to the individual patient and to the society that one serves.

CHAPTER VII

Team Practice

ONE OF PSYCHIATRY'S most important contributions to the art and science of medicine, in an age of increasing specialization and fragmentation of care, has been an emphasis on understanding the whole man, physical and mental, in his total environment. Our profession has taken a decidedly generalist stance in the face of increasing technology and specialization.

Community mental health program directors have tried to achieve the specialist's refined interest, study, and practice, without surrendering the superordinate goal of continuity of care, best served by a generalist all-purpose mode of organization. In most centers, this goal has been mediated through multidisciplinary team organization.

Community mental health programs can be ranked along a continuum, those with a maximum degree of specialization (such as the child guidance clinic) at one end and those with a great degree of generality (such as the state hospital) at the other. Further, it appears that specialization can be maintained only by a high degree of exclusiveness in patient selection. High'y specialized facilities, in effect, route patients on "shopping tours," until the agency or clinic or practitioner serving their special problem can be found.

On the other hand, the generalist stance—all things to all men—is decidedly harder on staff, who are, after all, human beings with their own needs and limitations. The psychiatric supermarket tends to exhaust staff, to drive them away. Worse yet, it sanctions group delusions; certain patients can be turned away by labeling them "bad" or "unmotivated" or by giving them "disciplinary discharges," promising treatment when and if undesirable symptoms abate.

The clinician is faced, in most community mental health centers, then, with the need to reconcile the conflicting pressures of quantity with quality services. Community mental health centers try to develop organizational arrangements which will approach the ideal goal of totally comprehensive and continuous care within a context of real expectations and with staff of limited stamina, capacities, and skills. In this endeavor, the extreme of therapeutic grandiosity is as dangerous as its opposite pitfall, therapeutic nihilism.

In translating slogans and idealistic schemes into operational reality, mental health center directors try to follow the guide of pragmatic Utopianism: achieve the attainable and pursue the ideal. Easy but limited success is not enough. Neither is imperfection cause for dismay. Progress is a series of successive approximations of the desired state.

Perhaps the Denver experience can serve as a useful guide for what may be ahead for those mental health practitioners entering the community mental health center system. In setting up the comprehensive mental health program in Denver, we wished to have the advantages of functional team organization; we wanted our staff divided into small social groupings, each with a defined role and leadership structure. Literature in both social psychology and business management gives evidence that such organization is overwhelmingly favored. In line with our knowledge of effective group functioning, we wanted to keep the teams small. While we wanted an organization with clear leadership and authority structure, we also wanted to allow maximum freedom for all disciplines to expand their functional roles.

We also desired an organization which would facilitate comprehensive and continuous care. From the experience of other "innovative" programs, we knew that attempting to load a team with undivided responsibility for total care for all patients could result in the adoption of relatively rigid, stereotyped, and ritualized approach to patients, attempting to fit all of them into the standard treatment modality. If the team should feel incapable of meeting the needs of a particular patient, it could be tempted to define him as resistant or unsuitable. We wished to provide, then, a system of internal echelons with backup or specialized resources available to each outpatient team to supplement and complement the comprehensive and continuous care that they, the "generalist" teams, offered.

We particularly did not want to discard hard-won

insights of behavioral science practitioners, gained over the last several decades. We did not want to substitute an entirely new orthodoxy of therapeutic community, community psychiatry, mental health consultation, or any other "bold new approach" for the older rigid belief systems. We *did* want to develop a system that is eclectic, patient-centered, task-oriented, and organized to facilitate clinical problem-solving. The basic theses of our program are summarized in Figure 1.

The organization that evolved from these desires and convictions is based on a functional group called the generic mental health team. The crux of our program consists of six generic teams which operate as psychiatric general practitioners, serving defined geographic areas with populations between 45,000 and 90,000. The generic teams are charged with providing readily available care. Their primary responsibility is continuity of care, monitoring the longitudinal treatment course of each patient whether he is receiving treatment from that team, the psychiatric hospital service, other backup resource, or some other facility. Terminal outpatient treatment and restoration to nonpatient status is the responsibility of the generic team.

While Denver is not functionally organized along geographic lines, and while there are many disadvantages and artificialities in utilizing a geographic model, we felt it was the most efficient approach at this phase in developing the comprehensive community mental health program. All of the teams are currently in clinic or office facilities within their service areas.

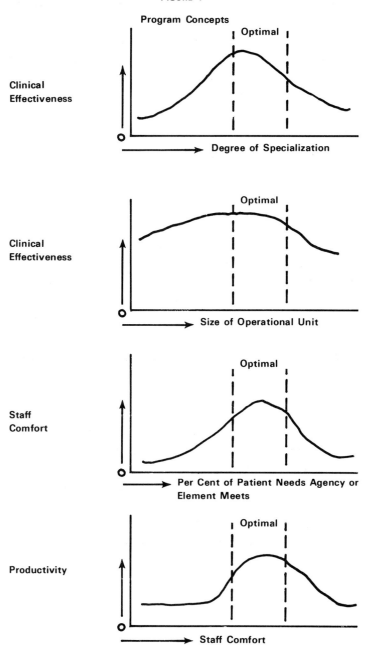

FIGURE 1

Within its geographic service area, each generic team is responsible for developing a comprehensive mental health program, calling on centralized or backup resources to complement the services the team provides directly. The tasks such a team confront in developing this program for its service area, according to our experience, may be summarized this way:

Know the Service Area

The service areas in all cities have widely differing characteristics. First, demographic characteristics of different portions of the city are variable. Age, ethnicity, education, and socioeconomic distribution are only a few of the population traits which should be studied.

Second, the area may be the locus of a particular kind of problem, such as single-parent families or multiple boarding and nursing homes. An area with many children will obviously make different demands on its generic team than one with a predominantly aging population. The team will want to emphasize child psychiatric services and consultation to schools and other child-caring agencies for one; in the other, they might well focus on developing community resources to prevent desocialization and mental illness in older citizens.

There are a number of sources for such information. The most recent census data, while always out of date, is a good starting point. Additional data, particularly concerning the incidence of recognized social or personal pathology, is available from the state mental health authority. The community mental health center itself should develop centralized information concerning new admissions to both generic and specialized teams.

The Visiting Nurse Service is a very important source of information; individual Visiting Nurses have considerable experience and can give teams valuable, although subjective, information about the neighborhood. The Department of Welfare also has current data concerning socioeconomic characteristics of clients, by census tract. Police records, juvenile court records, county and district court records provide information about the prevalence and types of socially disordered behavior which are matters of public concern in the area.

After compilation, this information should be the basis for planning services to meet the needs of the area. Individuation of the team's program is, in most centers, left to the initiative and authority of the team leader. One of the strengths of the team-organized and decentralized program is that it allows great latitude for initiative in developing unique and desirable programs.

Develop a Problem-Solving and Supervisory System

The team must develop its own internal ground rules for approaching its superordinate goals; otherwise, internal conflicts, dissension, and inefficiency will prevail. Social and psychological research has clearly demonstrated that problem-solving mechanisms must be evolved for healthy and efficient small group functioning.

There are a number of methods by which the internal control and regulation system can be established and sustained. The team leader's direct supervision of the clinical work of all team members is an important aspect of internal control. He should meet individually with each team member at least once a week. He should also review, at least once each quarter, the entire careload of each team member.

Team meetings, at least twice weekly, are another important part of the team's social control system. They provide the means for mutual support, for professional development of newer team members, for correction of counter-transference distortion, and for sharing responsibility among team members. Weekly case conferences with consultants assigned in rotation, and consultation from staff supervisors in nursing and social work, are other elements of team problem-solving.

An adequate record-keeping system is a vital element of effective and responsible social control. Such records are reviewed for periodic team evaluation by special committees, and the record-keeping forms are continually revised with the intent of developing a quality control and program evaluation system throughout all functional elements of the Division of Psychiatric Services.

Approximately 15 per cent of total team time is devoted to communication, problem-solving, consultation, supervision, and record-keeping.

Develop a Good Clinical Program

The clinical program of the generic mental health team must have certain minimal elements: availability, comprehensiveness, continuity and quality of care.

To help achieve *availability,* teams should be decentralized into their service areas. The team will usually be charged with seeing all patients—both adults and children with all types and degrees of illnesses—as soon as possible; preferably, on the day of initial inquiry. Any one of the team members may serve as the primary clinician conducting the evaluation, and he is expected to adopt a family orientation. Family therapy is not the treatment of choice for many patients, but the initial evaluation procedure should be family-oriented.

The generic team should also attempt to answer all needs for emergency evaluations, calling on other psychiatric emergency services only when its own resources are exhausted. All generic teams should have evening or Saturday hours, and all are responsible for facilitating improved communication with other agencies and caregivers in the area to increase the availability of their service.

Comprehensiveness of care envisions each team providing a full spectrum of outpatient services, ranging from individual counseling and casework to prolonged individual psychotherapy, family therapy, and sociotherapy. Large and small group therapy options should run the gamut in terms of demand, expressiveness, goals, duration, and focus. Groups should range between small group psychotherapy sessions, traveling and activity therapy groups for children, marital partner groups, and large social hours. Chemotherapy must be utilized intelligently, never relegating those patients receiving medication to the role of second-class citizens in our clinical program.

Since generic teams cannot and should not develop all elements of comprehensive mental health services for their areas, specialized resources exist in most community mental health centers to complement and augment the treatment modalities available at the generic team level.

Continuity of care is attempted at all program levels. The same clinician on the generic team assumes primary responsibility for initial evaluation, treatment, and follow-up of the patient whenever possible. Generic team members may participate in rounds and staff planning conferences for their patients on the hospital service; they may also conduct small group therapy sessions with their hospitalized patients, with a hospital staff member as co-therapist. Generic teams should also be encouraged to maintain regular contact, often through a series of informal meetings, with their counterparts at the state hospital and various voluntary and United Fund agencies, to enhance continuity of care for patients whose needs are not met by any single agency.

Quality control is difficult to achieve at this stage of the art in psychiatry. The team leader bears primary responsibility, administratively, ethically and legally, for developing and maintaining high standards of clinical care. He is responsible for direct supervision of clinical activities of all his team members, both individually and as a group. His own efforts must be enhanced by utilization of specialty consultation or supervision, mandatory for social workers without ACSW accreditation and any other team members for whom such supervision is felt to be necessary. Weekly all-staff conferences, case conferences, and inservice training programs constitute other efforts of most community mental health centers to improve quality by continually upgrading staff competence.

The typical generic team might be expected to absorb a clinical load of eight to 10 new patients a week, or 400 to 500 new patients in a year. It is anticipated that about half would be seen in individual psychotherapy for a mean number of seven appointments. About one-fourth of the caseload would be treated in group therapy, with an approximate mean number of 30 sessions. The remaining one-fourth of the patients would fall into a wide variety of treatment categories.

It is estimated that generic teams should initially devote about 50 per cent of total team hours to direct clinical services (15 per cent for evaluation, 15 per cent for individual treatment, 20 per cent for group therapy), with an additional 15 per cent for treatment and preventive activities for alcoholics. As the team matures, the percentage of team time devoted to direct clinical services would be anticipated to decrease to approximately 40 per cent.

Develop a Mental Health Consultation Program

The generic mental health team is expected to provide two types of consultative services for other agencies and caregivers in its area: Formal consultation sessions should be regularly scheduled, at least once a month, for staff groups from other agencies; informal consultation should be available as needed, often over the telephone, to help individual caregivers deal with specific client problems.

There are many reasons for developing a good consultation program. First, it allows the team to get a much fuller and more realistic grasp of community needs and problems. Second, consultation with primary sources of referral allows the team some control on timing and some selection over the types of referrals. Consultation also helps other agencies to provide increasingly effective mental health care, and it improves their casefinding and referral abilities, which have impact in the area of prevention. A well-developed consultation program promotes good will and interagency cooperation and builds a backlog of "social credit" for the team with other agencies in its area.

The typical steps in developing an ongoing consultation program involve first obtaining top-level sanction from the administrator of the agency approached. After obtaining his approval, a plan and goals for the consultation process should be developed with him and/or his designatee. This plan should include a structure for regular visits by a specified team member or members and guidelines for the consultees. Confidential issues should be dealt with, and provisions should be made for periodic evaluation between consultants, team leader, and director and consultees of the agency.

The typical team initially devotes about 10 per cent of total time to consultation, gradually increasing consultative services to 25 per cent of team time. With the development of two additional comprehensive mental health centers to serve the presently unserved portions of Denver, it is anticipated that the clinical caseload of generic teams will decrease and consultation will occupy up to half of the total team time.

Develop Community Organization and Public Education Programs

If the community mental health center is indeed to continue as a trusted and valued member of the helping community, it must develop a broad base of public understanding, support, and mutual assistance within each team service area. Developing this community sanction cannot be done only by the director of the mental health center or a few staff members. It must be accomplished by every staff member throughout the community, every day. Ignoring this aspect of community mental health practice means that our program will falter and may fail when the going gets rough.

Our knowledge about community organization in an urban area is limited, at best. By approaching the task at the generic team level, however, there are several ways to organize local support. A generic team may constitute two kinds of community groups. The first is a citizens advisory council, broadly representative of various vested interest groups in the area, such as the ministerial alliance, the Chamber of Commerce, the mental health association, neighborhood action agencies of the war on poverty, and others. The purpose of this group is to help the team elicit broad community support, to keep the team informed of community sentiment and needs, and to help the team plan needed mental health programs and services. The second group is a community resources council, representing major social and health agencies and professions in the area, formed primarily to plan interagency services for multiple-problem families.

The consultation program is probably the single most effective tool for developing a broad base of community understanding and support. In addition to team time allotted for structured consultation, at least five per cent of total time should be devoted to other community organization and public education activities. Availability for public speaking in the team service area is another extremely useful way of making the team known to its constituents.

Develop Special Projects

There are a number of projects which can be developed, once basic team goals are achieved, to meet special needs of the area, and which are suited to the interests of staff members. Specialized services to nursing and boarding homes, preventive programs in public housing projects or housing development areas, preventive intervention in families with pending divorce actions or with adolescent runaways, a variety of school-related projects, workshops and seminars for ministers or general practitioners have been developed in Denver by the generic health teams, as they have been in other communities by other agencies. Up to five per cent of total team time may be devoted to such special projects.

Develop Training Potential

Generic mental health teams may provide fieldwork experience for students and trainees in the wide spectrum of mental health professions: psychiatric interns and residents, psychology interns, social work students (casework, groupwork, and community organization), graduate students in psychiatric nursing, special education students, and graduate students in rehabilitation.

This assumption of training responsibility is vital for personal and professional development of team members and for long-range contribution to the community and professions. Every team member needs a genuine commitment to training, in addition to the discipline provided in clinical experience. For every hour of clinical staff supervision, at least three hours of trainee direct service will probably be expected.

Develop Research and Scientific Publication Activities

At the present stage of development of community psychiatry, clear basic program descriptions are very helpful to other practitioners. An honest and thoughtful description of a program and its apparent impact is in no way to be sneered at or downgraded in terms of its usefulness to program planners. Attempts at systematic evaluation of program modifications, such as changes in patient caseload when a generic team moves out of the hospital, are needed. Treatment outcome research is probably the most difficult; that and basic research should be undertaken only with major commitment to planning, large amounts of time, and additional staff and/or financial support.

The average community psychiatric team provides this spectrum of community services with approximately 340 manhours a week, if the full potential of all team members is utilized. The "typical team" consists of a psychiatrist, a clinical psychologist, two psychiatric social workers, a psychiatric nurse, a half-time rehabilitation counselor, clinicians (in any discipline) with experience in the treatment of alcoholics and children, a secretary-receptionist, students and trainees, and about four subprofessional members, either volunteers or indigenous neighborhood aides.

When we set up this organizational system in Denver early in 1966, we subdivided the existing outpatient department into the nuclei of teams, subsequently adding personnel. The old child guidance clinic was abolished, and those personnel were reassigned to the generic teams. On each team there is now a degree of internal specilization; some staff members prefer to work with children, others are skilled with chronic psychotic patients, with adolescents, and so forth.

One of management's responsibilities in assigning personnel to the teams is not only to assess the personal compatability of team members, but also to balance their professional strengths and weaknesses so a functional working unit can evolve. While objective guidelines for this assessment are not available, it is a traditional function of administration and has crucial importance in determining the effective operation of the team unit.

THE SPECIALIZED SERVICES

The generic mental health teams are not expected to directly provide total comprehensive care to patients in their districts; a second echelon of specialized services must be available within the organizational system for the generic teams to call upon as needed. In requesting assistance from these specialized resources, the generic team should not rid itself of responsibility for the patient; rather, it calls in temporary assistance to extend needed services to individual patients. Responsibility for monitoring the patient's course of treatment and for providing continuing outpatient treatment remain with the generic team. The specialized services available to the generic teams in Denver are briefly detailed below.

The Psychiatric Hospital Service

The hospital services team operates a combined inpatient and day hospital treatment program, essentially an open therapeutic community. The generic team psychiatrist may admit patients to the hospital service himself for either 24-hour or day treatment. With only 16 inpatient beds and a capacity of 24 in the day program, hospital stay is very brief; it averages about one week for inpatients, about three weeks for day patients.

The generic team participates in hospital grand rounds to discuss treatment course and posthospital planning for patients from its service area; it also helps conduct small group therapy for hospitalized patients from the area. This outpatient participation in hospital activities is essential to continuity of care. It also provides good inservice training for hospital nurses who serve as co-therapists for small groups, and it facilitates communication between outpatient and hospital staffs.

The Visiting Nurse Service

In Denver, the Visiting Nurse Service is part of the public health program of the Department of Health and Hospitals. Visiting Nurses supply not only traditional home nursing services, but are frequently requested to follow a patient who has missed an appointment or to make an evaluative home visit to extend team understanding of an adult or child problem. In the first six months of 1968, Visiting Nurses made 2,740 home evaluative or therapeutic visits at the request of generic teams. Two specialized Visiting Nurses are assigned full-time to boarding and nursing homes housing psychiatric patients and conduct weekly group counseling sessions there with generic team members as cotherapists.

Children's Services

Each generic team has a part- or full-time member with training and experience in the treatment of children, so that comprehensive services for children are available at the neighborhood level. However, we do not expect the teams to have full competence in such areas of child psychiatry as differential diagnosis of the minimally brain-damaged child, treatment of autistic and schizophrenic children, and so forth. A small child psychiatric staff, which is operationally part of the neighborhood health program of the Department of Health and Hospitals, furnished consultation to the generic teams, the pediatrics service of Denver General Hospital, and other child-caring agencies in Denver. This team also operates specialized treatment facilities, such as a diagnostic and therapeutic nursery for preschool children, and a psychoeducational program for brain-damaged and perceptually handicapped children, which are referral sources for the generic teams.

Medical Services

A full-time general practitioner provides physical examinations and any other medical services desired by the generic teams. For some teams, the physician has primary medical responsibility for patients in the alcoholism treatment program, and he conducts medication clinics, with a nonpsychiatrist team member, for chronically ill patients.

Rehabilitation Services

In addition to the services of a half-time rehabilitation counselor on each generic mental health team, a centralized rehabilitation program is available for patients who have major problems in achieving and maintaining adequate social, vocational, and educational adjustment.

Psychological Testing Laboratory

One of the primary goals of community psychiatry is to make treatment more economically available. The psychological testing laboratory supplies group-administered screening batteries to patients, both adult and child, referred by generic mental health teams. Teams may also refer patients for individual tests administered by a psychometrician. Test data are routinely submitted to the generic team psychologist for his interpretation in expanding the team's understanding of the patient.

Psychiatric Emergency Service

About 200 patients each month are evaluated and provided psychiatric first aid by the psychiatric emergency team, staffed primarily by psychiatric nurses. The team is on duty, in shifts, 18 hours a day in the emergency room of Denver General Hospital. In addition to its direct clinical services in the emergency room, the team operates a telephone suicide prevention service and follows attempted suicides who are hospitalized at Denver General Hospital. The team requests home visits from Visiting Nurses for suicide attempters who are sent home after emergency medical treatment and for women who come to the emergency room after a sexual assault.

About one-third of the patients seen by the psychiatric emergency team are referred to another community agency, such as Fort Logan Mental Health Center, the V. A. Hospital, or a private practitioner of psychiatry. Others are referred to the psychiatric hospital service or the appropriate generic mental health team; some are carried directly by the emergency team in short-term crisis therapy.

Training and Education

A problem of the decentralized program is maintaining commonality of purpose and preventing fragmentation. An antidote is a strong agency-wide inservice training program which brings various professions from the functional units together. The inservice training program of the Division of Psychiatry has ongoing discussion seminars, attended by personnel from all teams according to their interests and learning needs in community psychiatry, family therapy, group therapy, crisis intervention, behavior therapy, and other topics of current interest. About every three months, we have a special workshop in an area of general interest to all staff, such as alcoholism, aftercare, forensic psychiatry, consultation, and so forth.

CONCLUSION

There is no magic or outstanding wisdom in this organizational structure of the Division of Psychiatry. The means of combining generalist and specialist approaches are well-known organizational principles that have been used for centuries in industry, education, warfare, and government. This plan, like any other, will succeed or fail depending on the commitment and energy invested in it by people in leadership and authority roles throughout the system. The example they set determines, in large part, the operation of the program. While it is too soon to tell with certainty, this pattern of service—decentralized generic teams backed up by centralized specialty service—appears to be the pattern for most effectively developing community mental health services. In such a setting, then, the practitioner may expect to apply the clinical skills discussed in previous chapters. Obviously, new role stresses, as well as new opportunities, abound in such an organization. Until more practitioners receive a percentage of their training in this kind of setting, new staff members will have problems adapting.

FIGURE 2

Tasks of the Generic Mental Health Team

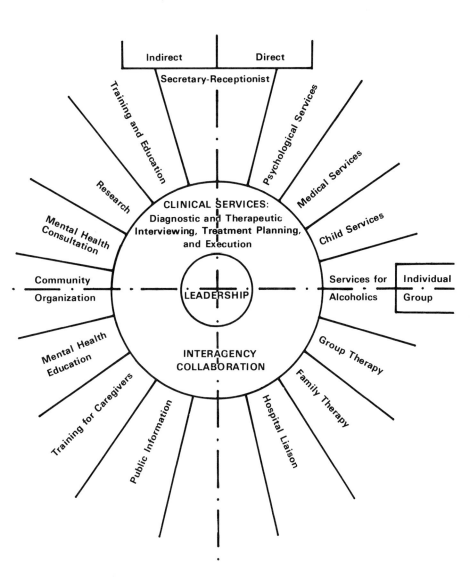

CHAPTER VIII

Recapitulation: Expectations and Opportunities

THE PRECEDING chapters have detailed some of the unique characteristics of clinical practice in comprehensive community mental health settings. In the process, it was hopefully made clear that this new social institution, the comprehensive community mental health center, establishes new demands on our mental health practitioners, as well as opening up new opportunities. Those of us already in the field must modify our behavior to respond to those challenges, and training centers must increase their competency to assist trainees to expand their role definition and enhance their role competency. Let us highlight some of the expectations of a community mental health practitioner:

1. His self-identity is that of a decision-maker and a problem-solver, not primarily a psychotherapist, a psychopharmacologist, etc. He defines his adequacy in terms of the relevance of his functioning to the life dilemmas presented by the clients of a comprehensive community mental health program. He bases his self-esteem not primarily on his technical

competence in a defined change technology, but rather his ability to understand the problems that his client faces, and to bring to bear optimal change technology.

2. He sees his contribution as part of a general system addressed to the problems of individuals and of the community as a whole. He attempts to transcend the focus that he has, as a clinician, upon the individual patient and to understand his function within a larger and more complex social system which has been set up to respond to needs defined by the larger community. Consequently, he accepts the desirability of, and hopefully enthusiastically supports, program evaluation and research, which studies therapeutic transactions within the context of the community mental health center system.

3. The practitioner finds himself functioning as a booking agent or broker, a task for which he usually has received no specific training in his professional education. If he assesses the needs of his clients honestly and comprehensively, he recognizes that no single practitioner can master all of the available intervention strategies useful to certain individuals. Consequently, he—as the private physician has been doing unwittingly in this country for years—serves as a purchasing agent, helping his patient find and gain access to needed services. In this process, he must address himself not only to appropriateness and availability of service, but also to continuity and comprehensiveness of care. He serves as a representative, then, of a community mental health system, and of the larger social system of his community, which has a number of alternatives for

assisting individuals with deviant thoughts, feelings, and behaviors.

4. He is unalterably a team worker. Because the practitioner recognizes the complexity of patient needs and the range of applicable change technology, he has accepted the necessity of working as a member of a multidisciplinary staff in order that his patients and society may be more adequately served. This exposes him to status and hierarchical problems as well as role pressures and tensions he often was not prepared for by an esoteric and isolated training program.

5. He maintains a firm grasp on reality, appraising his own functioning, the system's, and the needs of his patients. He is a pragmatic Utopian, living with the existential anguish that is inescapable when one honestly confronts the inequalities, pressures, and hazards of the real world. He is leery of idealistic schemes, of simplistic solutions to the dilemmas of the human condition, and of exclusivistic systems of belief and practice.

6. He is cognizant of his public responsibility, and considers himself a public servant. He soon discovers that the public servant is regarded ambivalently by the nutrient culture, and that he must endure and somehow cope with the frequent "put downs" of his colleagues in private practice, and of many individuals in our society who are still wedded to an exploitative, materialistic, money-oriented point of view. Early in his career in a comprehensive community mental health center, he must decide whether he can gain sufficient gratification from the outcome of his practice, his association with colleagues and

peers within the community mental health center, and his sense of having implemented his belief system vigorously through his own life; or whether he requires the rewards of fame, status in the community, and money which would await him in the private sector.

This book highlights the flux, the excitement, and the change inherent in the community mental health center movement in the United States today. A handful of visionary pragmatists set about to move our nation from the worst public mental health service delivery system in the civilized world to the best. In doing so, the belief systems of free enterprise are challenged, and the startling proposal is made that public services are capable of equaling if not exceeding in quality those deployed by the private sector. Many individual practitioners who have chosen to commit themselves to the community mental health center concept, and who have risen to leadership positions, are consequently committed not only to an improvement in the clinical service available to American citizens, but also to helping our society escape its chauvinistic devotion to capitalistic free enterprise as an inherently superior system of accomplishing national goals. Government is not the enemy of our citizens, nor is society the enemy of the individual. Large sectors of the American mental health establishment are still fixated at the simplistic view of man and his society expounded by Sigmund Freud in some of his early writings. At that time, Freud, with considerable justification, viewed the group, society, and community as the enemy of the individual. In the hierarchical, stratified, rigid, and privilege-ridden society of which he was a member, there was much supportable evidence for this point of view. The events leading up to World War I, and the period during and subsequent to that terrible upheaval, further heightened Freud's consciousness of the tension between the individual and society.

Many of us in community psychiatry today are trying to escape from a naive view of man and are rejecting the dichotomization of the rights and needs of the individual and the rights and needs of the culture of which he is a member. That a certain tension exists is undeniable. It has existed from the days of the earliest tribes; it is clearly documented in the Old Testament of the Bible; it is spelled out in elaborate detail, often punctuated with blood, in the history of our own country. It is demonstrated daily in our urban riots, in the protests of students on our campuses, in the attack on many of the cherished norms and institutional forms of our American society.

It is an integral part of the American dream, a part of the American conviction, a part of the history of American progress, that society can be made to more closely approximate the needs, and to facilitate the aspirations, of its individual members. A fatalism that proclaims an eternal and unremitting enmity between society and the individual is unworthy of us as scientists, and unbefitting us as Americans. The American dream is that government can and must serve the people, that individual liberty must be preserved and the right to dissent shall be safeguarded, and that the pressures of religious and other exclusivistic belief systems not be allowed to dominate the lives of individual citizens. Those of us in community mental health believe that it is quite possible to stand at the interface between the individual and his society and to serve both fairly, effectively, nonrepressively, and honestly.

Society cannot exist without men. Nor can men, if the history of human events is to be taken seriously, live without society.

In this book, the author has attempted to focus on one of the many threads in community mental health practice: the clinical function. The emphasis on identification, treatment, and rehabilitation of the adaptational casualty is most congruent with the clinical and humanistic tradition of the mental health disciplines. It is a job we must do well, not only because of any inherent good in that process, but also because it gives us an entry into the lives of individuals and of the community, allowing us to understand the need for preventive mental health services and to more fully conceptualize the points of leverage and the processes that will be necessary to reduce the incidence of adaptational casualties in our communities. The clinician and preventive mental health worker may or may not be combined in the same professional person, but at any event they have a shared destiny and a common purpose: the betterment of the quality of human life in this time for the people of the United States.

Bibliography

Bellak, L. & Barten, H. H., eds. (1969), *Progress in Community Mental Health,* Vol. I. New York: Grune & Stratton.

Berne, E. (1964), *Games People Play.* New York: Grove Press.

Brodsky, C. M., Fischer, A., & Wilson, G. C. (1969), Analysis of a treatment-decision system. *Dis. Nev. Supt.,* 30:17–23.

Glasscote, R. M., Gudeman, J. E., et al. (1969), *The Staff of the Mental Health Center: A Field Study.* Washington, D.C.: The Joint Information Service.

_____ Craft, A. M., Glassman, S. M., & Jepson, W. W. (1969), *Partial Hospitalization for the Mentally Ill.* Washington, D.C.: The Joint Information Service.

_____ Sussex, J. N., Cumming, E., & Smith, L. H. (1969), *The Community Mental Health Center, An Interim Appraisal.* Washington, D.C.: The Joint Information Service.

_____ Plaut, T. F. A., Hammersley, D. W., O'Neill, F. J., Chafetz, M. E., & Cumming, E. (1967), *The Treatment of Alcoholism.* Washington, D.C.: The Joint Information Service.

Halleck, S. (1967), *Psychiatry and the Dilemmas of Crime.* New York: Harper & Row.

Heller, A., Zahourek, R., & Whittington, H. G. (1970), *A Triple Blind Comparison of Imipramine, Desipramine, and Placebo.* Manuscript.

Hornstra, R. K. & Wilkinson, C. B. (1966), Response of patients to termination of treatment in an aftercare clinic. *Arch. Gen. Psychiat.,* 14:644–650.

Jacobson, J. G. & Whittington, H. G. (1960), A study of process in the evaluation interview. *Psychiatry,* 23:23-44.

Joint Commission on Mental Illness and Health (1961), *Action for Mental Health.* New York: Basic Books.

Jones, M. (1962), *Social Psychiatry.* Springfield, Ill.: Charles C. Thomas.

Kennedy, J. F. (1964), Message from the President of the United States related to mental illness and mental retardation. *Amer. J. Psychiat.,* 120:729–737.

Langsley, D. G. & Kaplan, D. M. (1968), *The Treatment of Families in Crisis.* New York: Grune & Stratton.

May, P. R. (1968), *Treatment of Schizophrenia.* New York: Science House.

Menninger, K. A. (1962), *A Manual for Psychiatric Case Study.* New York: Grune & Stratton.

Padula, H., et al. (1968), *Approach to the Care of Long-Term Mental Patients.* Washington, D.C.: The Joint Information Service.

Pasamanick, B., Scarpetti, F. R., & Dimitz, S. (1967), *Schizophrenics in the Community.* New York: Appleton-Century-Croft.

Riessman, F., Cohen, J., & Pearl, A., eds. (1964), *Mental Health of the Poor.* New York: Free Press.

Ruesch, J. (1969), The assessment of social disability. *Arch. Gen. Psychiat.,* 21:655–664.

Shore, M. F. & Mannino, F. V., eds. (1969), *Mental Health and the Community: Problems, Programs, and Strategies.* New York: Behavioral Publications.

Whittington, H. G. (1963), *Psychiatry on the College Campus.* New York: International Universities Press.

———— (1966), *Psychiatry in the American Community.* New York: International Universities Press.

———— Zahourek, R., & Grey, L. (1969), Pharmacotherapy and community psychiatric practice. *Amer. J. Psychiat.,* 126:551–554.